The Ethics of
Environmentally Responsible
Health Care

The Ethics of Environmentally Responsible Health Care

Jessica Pierce
Andrew Jameton

OXFORD
UNIVERSITY PRESS
2004

OXFORD
UNIVERSITY PRESS

Oxford   New York
Auckland   Bangkok   Buenos Aires   Cape Town   Chennai
Dar es Salaam   Delhi   Hong Kong   Istanbul   Karachi   Kolkata
Kuala Lumpur   Madrid   Melbourne   Mexico City   Mumbai   Nairobi
São Paulo   Shanghai   Taipei   Tokyo   Toronto

Copyright © 2004 by Oxford University Press, Inc.

Published by Oxford University Press, Inc.
198 Madison Avenue, New York, New York, 10016

http://www.oup-usa.org

Oxford is a registered trademark of Oxford University Press

Library of Congress Cataloging-in-Publication Data
Pierce, Jessica, 1965-
The ethics of environmentally responsible health care/
Jessica Pierce, Andrew Jameton
p. cm.   Includes bibliographical references and index.
ISBN 0-19-513903-8 (cloth)
1. Medical ethics.   2. Environmental health—Moral and ethical aspects.
3. Bioethics.   4. Environmentally induced diseases—Moral and ethical aspects.
I. Jameton, Andrew.   II. Title.
R725.5.P547 2004   174'.2—dc21   2003042901

9 8 7 6 5 4 3 2 1

Printed in the United States of America
on recycled, acid-free paper
using soy-based ink

Preface

Our feeling for nature is like the feeling of an invalid for health.
—Friedrich Schiller, *On Naïve and Sentimental Poetry*, 1795–96

Bioethics originally encompassed both ecological and clinical concerns (Potter 1971), but almost immediately separated into distinct disciplines: bioethics, concerned with clinical practice, and environmental ethics. Though the fields still share a common philosophical foundation, they are profoundly disconnected in their practical concerns (Whitehouse 1999).

Health-care ethics zooms in on individual patients and their caregivers; environmental ethics deals in large populations, human and nonhuman. Clinical ethics episodes are usually resolved in days, weeks, or months; ecologists and environmental philosophers reflect on decisions and policies that play out over decades, centuries, and even millennia. Typically working in large medical centers amply supplied with skilled personnel, ingenious devices, and complex therapies, health-care ethicists tend to be optimistic about the value of new and complex technologies and the ability of ethical principles to manage potential difficulties. Environmentalists, who serve among the witnesses to widespread human poverty, increasing toxicity, and disappearing biodiversity, tend to be skeptical about the potential of new technology to solve human problems. The values and concerns of the two fields differ: health-care ethicists focus on autonomy, advocacy, clinical benefits, avoiding harm to patients, and fairness in limiting costs. Environmental philosophers consider such values as sustainability, ecosystem integrity, global interconnection, limits to growth, and respect for nature.

Can these two fields, so similar in their philosophical foundations and so different in their vocabulary and issues, be grasped in a unified way? There are good reasons to view the two fields as interconnected: High quality, ethically sound health care can survive only if the larger environment survives and sustains health. As individuals with integrity, we cannot safely separate our concern for the world from our daily lives. If we are to make sound ethical judgments in health care, we need to consider the environmental implications of our decisions.

How then should clinicians and health-care ethicists take into account the grim global context outside health care that environmental ethicists are so concerned about? What concepts from environmental ethics can be applied to health care, and how can they he combined with more traditional health-care ethics concepts? What kinds of case studies in health care highlight both clinical and environmental principles? What sorts of activities and responsibilities among clinicians and hospital administrators express an environmental awareness? What sorts of problems and obstacles, both theoretical and practical, stand in the way of environmentally sound health care practice?

Environmental principles are central to a responsibly inclusive understanding of bioethics and conduct of health care. Our argument for this is threefold:

First, environmentalism carries a clear and distressing message about the state of the earth's ecosystem and the prospects for life during the next few centuries. If the warnings of environmental scientists continue to go unheeded, the fate of humanity is bound to be dismal. Already, a substantial portion of earth's population is living in great poverty, and if more suffering from environmental decline is to be avoided, significant measures need to be taken to limit both population and consumption, primarily by the wealthiest sector of the world's population. Unless the human burden on the biosphere is relieved, expensive health-care technologies cannot eliminate disease and suffering.

Second, health care itself imposes significant environmental costs that can be reduced without harm to public health. Although the toxicity of health-care practices is the most commonly addressed of these costs in the United States, health care has a problem of overscale as well. Clinicians and ethicists need to take a wider view of clinical technologies that includes their environmental costs throughout their full life cycle of production, use, and disposal. Some health occupations already accept a responsibility for the stewardship of resources, but every health profession needs to accept responsibility for reducing the environmental impact of its services.

Third, design concepts and principles that are readily found in environmental and ecological thinking can be applied fruitfully to health-care practice. Yet ethical dilemmas arise in balancing advocacy for patients with stewardship of environmental resources. Reflection on these dilemmas in turn fosters a reinterpretation of common principles used in health-care ethics—such as autonomy, beneficence, avoiding harm, and justice—in the light of environmental concerns.

A common criticism of drafts of this book has been that it is "too idealistic," by which we fear readers mean "unrealistic." Indeed, if our reader's sense of healthfulness and personal abundance depends on a belief that the world still offers unlimited potential for material growth, then our work is unlikely to foster conviction. But everyone, and especially the world's wealthiest—that is, the 20% of the world who use 90% of the world's health-care resources (World Bank 1993)—needs to realize that the earth's limits are real. Personal abundance can depend neither ethically nor in fact on increased use of materials and energy. Instead, our ideal of rescuing people from disease and suffering must work within an appreciation of the earth's limits.

Longmont, Colorado   J. P.
Omaha, Nebraska   A. J.

Acknowledgments

Since this book has been in process off and on for a decade, the list of people to whom we are indebted is long. We apologize to those who have helped us along the way whom we have neglected to mention here.

Much of our research was conducted with the generous support of The Greenwall Foundation, which has funded two cycles of research: "The Green Health Center Project" and "Exploring Bioethics Upstream." Thanks, in particular, to William Stubing for trusting in the value of our work during its infant stages and tolerating its slow fruition. We are particularly indebted to the two "green groups," who met at University of Nebraska Medical Center with the support of The Greenwall Foundation. The first group outlined and discussed the "manifesto" and principles of the Green Health Center described in chapter five: Jennifer Chesworth, Alan Diener, Michael Gillespie, Hollis Glaser, Reneé Irvin, Michael McCally, John McClain, Michael Pritchard, Christine Reed, Hollie Shaner, Dale Stover, Mary Ellen Uphoff, Susanna von Essen, Julia Walsh, and Lynne D. Willett.

Thank you also to those who worked on the "Exploring Bioethics Upstream" project that explored UNMC/NHS decision processes regarding environmental issues: Jean Amoura, Bruce Dvorak, Karen Falconer Al-Hindi, Michael Gillespie, Donald S. Leuenberger, Pamela McCright, Catherine McGuire Roussel, Kristine McVea, Keith Mueller, Terry Paulsen, Ron Schaefer, Barbara Stock, Dale Stover, Mary Ellen Uphoff, Susanna von Essen, and Susan Waggoner.

We owe gratitude to many staff and administrators at the University of Nebraska Medical Center and Nebraska Health System (UNMC/NHS). We would like to thank, in particular, Rick Boldt, in Facilities Management, for access to committees, and for a wealth of information about incinerators, recycling facilities, trashcans, and dedication to the job. We also especially appreciate the access to facilities, participation in committees, and information so generously provided by Joe Graham, Jackie Parmenter, Frank Pietrantoni, Michael Powell, Ronald Schaefer, Carla Snyder, Tom Strudl, and others. Thanks to James Anderson, chair of the department of Preventive and Societal Medicine at UNMC, for patient financial and professional support to both of us. Shireen Rajaram (University of Nebraska at Omaha) and Catherine McGuire Roussel (Joslyn Institute for Sustainable Design) co-authored some of the key papers of our project. Christina Kerby Kessinger has lent years of help as a research assistant and grant administrator and has provided valuable feedback on material in the book. Christina is responsible for the lion's share of work on a number of the case studies presented in the text. Angella Bowman composed and maintained the original project web page (*http://www. unmc.edu/green*). Sue Nardie helped with details of the text. Carmen Pirruccello has provided steady secretarial support.

We would like to acknowledge the contribution of our students over the years, especially summer students, who contributed ideas, research, and writing: David Mair, Andrew Page, Bruce R. Smith, and Colleen Svoboda. We also especially appreciate the participation and research help of students Chanel Helgason, Jane Handina Murigwa Kanchense, Jason Papenfuss, Janis Petzel, Anahita Rashidi, Patricia Sullivan, and Sarah Webber. Thank you to Steve Pergam and Gina Ramirez-Wilson for founding the Student Alliance for Global Health at UNMC.

Carolyn Raffensperger at Science and Environmental Health Network and Michael Lerner at Commonweal have provided significant leadership, resources, and community for conversation and ideas. Their combined efforts on the Blue Mountain Lake and the Ecological Medicine meetings were particularly important. In Chapter five, we borrow some of the language and principles of the February 2002 ecological medicine statement posted at *http://www.sehn.org* and authored by Nancy Myers, Kenny Ausubel, Davis Baltz, Janine M. Benyus, Charlotte Brody, Gary Cohen, Tracey Easthope, Kathy Gerwig, Tom Goldtooth, Louis J. Guillette, Jr., Andrew Jameton, John M. Last, Michael McCally, Laurie Monti, Gary Nabhan, Jonathan A. Patz, Carolyn Raffensperger, Eric Rasmussen, Satinath Sarangi, Ted Schettler, Julia Walsh, Mark Jerome Walters, Peter Warshall, and Michael Lerner.

We also received help from the Center for Rural Affairs (Wyatt Fraas, Martin and Linda Kleinschmit), City Sprouts (Katherine Brown and Nancy Williams), Health Care Without Harm (Charlotte Brody, Gary Cohen, and Jamie Harvie), the Healthy Building Network (Tom Lent), Joslyn Institute for Sustainable Design (Catherine McGuire Roussel and Cecil Steward), National Association of Physicians for the Environment (John Grupenhoff), The Nightingale Institute for Health and the Environment (Hollie Shaner and Glenn McRae), Partners in Health (Paul Farmer and Jim Kim), Physicians for Social Responsibility (Michael McCally and Robert Musil), and the environmental affinity groups of the International Association of Bioethics and the American Society for Bioethics and the Humanities.

Many colleagues and friends provided valuable feedback, inspiration, and ideas which helped to shape the text: Peter Adair, William Aiken, Virginia Aita, Rebecca Anderson, Tom Athanasiou, Paul Basch, Arthur and Nancy Bartlett, Margaret P. Battin, Solomon Benatar, Grazia Borrini-Feyerabend, Stephen Boyden, Donald A. Brown, John H. Bryant, Dan Callahan, Courtney Campbell, Paul Carrick, Jody Carrigan, Christine Cassel, Eric Chivian, Gary Comstock, Carl Cranor, Terry Davies, Ron Davis, Strachan Donnelley, Martin Donohoe, Alan Durning, Howard Frumkin, Jennifer Girod, Lynn Goldman, Sam Gorovitz, Carl Greiner, Sydney Halpern, Trevor Hancock, Barbara Heinzen, Warren Hern, Karen Falconer Al-Hindi, Bart Gruzalski, Steve Heilig, Robert K. Hitchcock, Rachelle Hollander, David Hoosen, Lisa Husmann, Wes Jackson, Robert R. Jacobs, Dale Jamieson, Derrick Jensen, Albert R. Jonsen, Eric Juengst, Allen Katz, Thomas Kelly, Chris Kiefer, Fred Kirschenmann, Kuang Yunfei, Thomasine Kushner, Steve Larrick, Margaret MacKenzie, Ruth Macklin, Anthony J. McMichael, Donella Meadows, Diane Meier, Frances Mendenhall, Carolyn Merchant, Carl Mitcham, Anuradha Mittal, Peter Montague, Andrew Moss, Richard Norgaard, Deborah Novak, Mary O'Brien, Tobie Olsan, Karen Olson, Stephen Packard, Jonathan Patz, Joan Penrod, Henry Perkins, Cheri Pies, Lisa Potter, Van Rensselaer Potter, Connie Price, Malcolm Potts, Ruth Purtilo, Ravi Rajan, Warren Reich, Leonard Rifas, Allan Rodger, John Ryan, Peter Sauer, Toby Schonfeld, Ted Schrecker, Richard R. Sharp, James and Sara Shull, Barry Smith, Margaret Topf, Ted Tsoukalas, William Vitek, Karen Warren, Laura Westra, Mary Terrell White, Peter Whitehouse, Jane Wigle, Dan Wikler, Richard Wilkinson, Mary Wilson, Gerald Winslow, and Rosalee Yeaworth.

Jeff House at Oxford has been wonderfully supportive, patient, and insightful. Thank you.

We would like to give special thanks to Roger Pierce for his generous support and constructive criticism throughout the process. Roger read and greatly helped clarify the text of the book through each of its five major drafts, and has read, all told, at least a hundred chapters over the years. Special thanks to Katherine Brown for her clear spiritual vision, patience, inspiration, and her keen sense of living with our contradictions on this small planet.

And, of course, we would like to acknowledge, and dedicate this book to our families. Jessica wishes to thank Chris for his loving patience, Sage for introducing a new perspective on the value of the future, and Roger and Alexandra for modeling courage and hard work. Andrew wishes to express particular gratitude to his grandparents, all gardeners who loved the quiet natural world of the Midwest, his parents—his mother a gardener, his father a loving critic—and his daughter Rachel Jameton, a green chemist.

We are also grateful to Ben Lee at Oxford University Press for championing the use of recycled paper and soy-based inks in printing this book. We are making a donation on behalf of this book to the Arbor Day Foundation, and to the cities of Omaha and Longmont for planting trees.

Contents

The Ethics of
Environmentally Responsible
Health Care

1

The Challenge of Environmental Responsibility

Signs of Trouble

The foundation of human health rests on healthy, stable ecosystems. Our biotic environment provides us with the fundamentals necessary for healthy lives—food, water, oxygen, warmth, light, and fuel. Earth's ecosystems also supply the raw materials for our health-care services. The global fraying of ecosystems has grave implications for our health and our ability to treat illnesses, now and in the future. Although health around the world improved on average over the last half century, it is likely that these gains will be lost if the environmental foundation for health continues to deteriorate.

Evidence accumulates daily that human health is suffering as ecosystems sicken. Billions of people already experience the effects of degraded environments. Lack of clean water for drinking, sanitation, and hygiene affects a third to half of the world's population and is responsible for seven percent of all death and disease globally. Two and a half million children die each year from diarrhea alone, the primary cause of which is water-borne microorganisms. Hundreds of millions suffer from hunger and malnutrition. Chemical agents, particularly in air pollution, are considered major factors in increased rates of bronchitis, heart disease, and cancers. The incidence of asthma is mushrooming. Certain forms of cancer are on the rise. The health of people all over the globe is diminished by exposure to toxic substances such as lead, mercury, arsenic, cadmium, and dioxin. As local and global ecosystems show increasing signs of stress, human health is likely to become far less stable and far more difficult to maintain.

As we show in Chapter 2, these challenges to health are clearly global in nature, and require a coordinated response. Climate is changing everywhere; so is the global distribution of nitrogen and other basic chemicals of life. Heedless of national boundaries, polluted air and water travel everywhere. We share oceans, atmosphere, and biodiversity.

The central explanation for our environmental predicament is, as we argue in Chapter 3, that humans are reaching the outer limits of population and material growth. The story of Easter Island serves as a metaphor and historical precedent for our current situation: as the people who had migrated to Easter Island around the fifth century prospered and their population grew, they stripped their tiny land of its natural resources and fell into a constant state of war over what was left. By the sixteenth century they had all but destroyed themselves (Ponting 1991, 1–7). The earth as a whole is now a small overcrowded island; there is ample reason to worry that we, too—all of humanity—are shaping, and can already discern, the trajectory of our own demise.

The dynamic combination of population size, resource consumption, and technology is putting tremendous strain on natural systems. The proportion of environmental change attributable to human impact compared to nature has increased vastly in recent centuries and at exponentially increasing rates. Clearance of forests, use of water, acquisition of the products of plant growth, occupation of land, pollution of water and air, and mining of the earth have all grown immensely and are substantially transforming the earth. Humans are now causing the greatest rate of species extinction since the disappearance of the dinosaurs. In 1700, the largest city in the world was Istanbul at 700,000 people; by 2050, a population roughly equal to the world's present 6.5 billion population is expected to live in cities alone. Industrial capacity has grown about 75 times since 1800. Since 1900, carbon dioxide emissions have grown 17 times and water use 9 times. These figures offer a proportionate sense of how dramatically the human relationship to the earth has changed in a very short time, and how unprecedented our situation is historically. The combination of the human economy and our population has clearly outgrown the capacity of the earth to heal itself (Wilson 1993; Vitousek 1994; Meyer 1996, 2, 23; McNeill 2001, 360; Wackernagel 2002; Brown, Gardner, and Halweil 1998, 43). It is well beyond reasonable debate that humans must come to terms with natural limits by curbing the growth of human population and altering basic modes of material production to reconcile human welfare with a thriving nature.

Health care is itself increasingly environmentally problematic. As we explain in Chapter 4, the materials and methods of health care contribute to pollution, add to global warming and ozone depletion, and rely on an extensive natural resource base—the extraction, manufacturing, and use of which incurs a significant environmental burden both locally and globally. This is partly a problem of scale. The United States maintains the world's largest health-care system, spending close to half of all the money spent in the world on health care. Maintaining such a large health-care system requires a large economy. That economy, however, is making a substantial contribution to the decline in the state of the world's environment. And environmental decline is in turn harming human health and creating more illnesses in need of treatment. As the need for health care increases, this already oversized health-care system, caught in this vicious positive feedback cycle, is likely to respond by growing and thereby continuing to further compound health problems. As such, health care frustrates its own practical and moral commitment to promote and maintain human health.

A more modest material and energy economy is critical to averting further ecological catastrophe. The necessary changes in modes of production in society at large will inevitably entail parallel changes in health-care technology and delivery.

We need not view these changes as losses. It is important to appreciate the positive potential of more environmentally sound health care in relation to the environmental crisis. Health-care systems will increasingly be called on to respond to environmentally related illness. Clearly, health professionals will need to learn more about the environmental basis of disease so that they can effectively diagnose and treat their patients. With a proper global commitment to reproductive health services, health care can play a key role in limiting population growth. It can play a crucial role in counseling and education about diet, environmentally caused disease, and healthy lifestyles. And health care can continue to offer—and can even strengthen—its significant psychological function of providing assurance, care, and hope to those who are ill or injured.

Sustainable Health and Health Care

To make such significant changes in our outlook on health care, we need to rethink the nature of health itself. In Chapter 5, we begin to describe a more ecological concept of health that reconciles and balances environmental, population, and individual health, and that orients human well-being toward greater respect for its dependency on the health of ecosystems.

A sustainable health perspective recognizes that the overall public health gains realizable from health care are limited. Allocating resources to meet the health-care needs of individuals should be framed in the context of maintaining sustainable public health for all people and ecosystems. Thus, a potentially unbounded investment in the rescue of the acutely ill and the treatment of the dying must be set aside to protect the resources necessary for prioritizing public health and prevention over health-care services. Fewer, more carefully chosen treatments and technologies may be offered, with an eye toward serving the key health needs of as many as possible, within global environmental constraints.

The move toward sustainable health care has the potential to resolve many problems of our current health-care system. Health care costs, disorganization, inaccessibility, side effects, mistakes, and disappointments are already at a high level; scaling health care down to a sustainable level can do much to heal many of these chronic health policy problems. Moreover, a sustainable health-care system permits a strong commitment to social justice in the United States. By reducing the material scale of health care, a sustainable system will, instead of lowering public health standards, support a higher level of access to health care and public health services for more people.

Sustainable health care recognizes that health is a global concern, which implies a strong principle of equality. We should seek to promote the environmental requirements of health (a healthy ecosystem, clean water, food, hygiene, and shelter), basic public health services (immunizations, reproductive health services, prenatal care), and modest health care for all, around the globe.

In addition to scaling down, sustainable health care can embody environmental values through design of buildings and grounds, choice of products, even the food served in the cafeteria. An increased appreciation of limits and of interconnection will affect what people value in health care.

Yet there are many practical and ethical issues involved in working toward a sustainable health-care system, one that is responsive to environmental limits and willing to reset priorities in order to balance good human health with ecological health (as there are many moral implications of choosing to ignore environmental limits). To explore the ethical principles of sustainable health in practice, we present in Chapter 5 the idea of the Green Health Center (GHC), a hypothetical health-care institution that embodies the values of sustainable health. The GHC would integrate environmental considerations into the design of its buildings, grounds, transportation systems, energy, and waste flows. The types of products and technologies used in the GHC would be evaluated with environmental costs in mind. The institution would offer a limited range of services and seek to provide adequate, efficient, and widely accessible care that is both economically and environmentally sustainable. The mission of the GHC is to demonstrate that sustainable health care is a feasible goal, both practically and morally, and to highlight areas of particular ethical concern.

In Chapters 5 and 6, we examine some of the specific moral tensions generated by taking environmental concerns seriously. We ask such questions as: Is environmental cost a legitimate factor to consider in weighing the clinical value of a particular treatment or technology? Should only those treatments be delivered that minimize environmental burden? Do physicians and other health professionals have role-specific responsibilities for environmental protection? Should human health on a societal or global scale be a significant concern for health professionals? Or, following the traditional reading of the Hippocratic oath, should clinicians serve only the individual?

Justice and Connection

In addition to raising local and specific questions about the nature of clinical services, a sustainable health perspective forces us to interpret these questions in a
broad global frame. In Chapter 7, we argue that U.S. health care cannot adequately
or ethically address human health or environmental preservation without appreciating health care's global interconnections. The resource base the health care
system is accustomed to draw on is essentially global. Disruption of global carbon and nitrogen cycles, loss of species, and pollution of air and oceans in other
regions of the world are likely to affect U.S. health care. Moreover, Americans
and others in consumption-heavy regions of the world are to some degree responsible for them. How those in the First World economies use resources to lead
meaningful lives, including providing themselves with health-care services, has
implications for the health of people in far-off places and in the future. What level
of responsibility do consumers have for the welfare of those far away? How should
Americans balance the health needs of U.S. citizens against the health needs of
people in other countries? And how does framing responsibility globally alter the
ethics conversation?

For many around the world, the proposal to embrace limits will seem like a cruel
joke: many people live on almost nothing, far less than the essentials for a decent
life. Limits on consumption must be primarily the responsibility of those who live
in abundance. This is a matter of both ecological necessity and justice. But choosing
to limit consumption and to lead simpler lives has implications for health policy.
Access among the wealthy to high-tech, environmentally costly services must be
seen, in a global context, as a low priority, incompatible with the need to share
health resources widely and efficiently. This means that universal access to health
care cannot be achieved sustainably by assuming wide access to existing health-
care technologies; instead, the technologies themselves will need to be redesigned.

One of the key insights grounding this book is borrowed from Herschel Elliott:
"An acceptable system of ethics is contingent on its ability to preserve the ecosystems that sustain it" (1997). Chapter 8 focuses on the work that bioethics itself
can do in supporting the move toward sustainable health. Bioethics can help establish an appreciation of limits and help make the transformation to modest consumption and a valuing of nature. Conventional principles of bioethics such as
nonmaleficence, respect for autonomy, and justice need to be reformulated in the
light of the changing global environment. And on some common issues in bioethics, different conclusions may be reached.

We strive here to bridge the gulf that separates environmental perspectives from
the viewpoints of health professionals and the ethicists in their midst. Millions of
people have been thinking about sustainability for a long time. Our book aims to
bring to the attention of clinical ethicists and health professionals years of work
by committed and concerned people trying to offer reflective solutions to what

seems to be a disaster in the making. We try to bring this careful thinking about the environmental crisis to bear on health care. Others are also working on this challenging translation and we hope that still more will join in the dialogue.

Environmental Trends in Medicine and Bioethics

Although medical care in the United States seems, on the whole, to be proceeding as if the sea change in the global environment were occurring on a different planet, there are also strong voices for reform. Beginning in the mid–twentieth century, some health professionals began expressing concern about the health implications of modern environmental decline (Berrill 1955; Schultz 1945). Especially in the past decade, interest in the environment–health connection has been growing.

Environmental health issues are increasingly appearing in the mainstream medical literature. Of particular note, the *Canadian Medical Association Journal* published in 2001 a series of articles on the environment and health. The series focused on the health effects of global warming, loss of biodiversity, stratospheric ozone depletion, consumption, toxic chemicals, pollution, population growth, and war (now collected in McCally 2002). Many of these concerns echo an earlier edited book entitled *Critical Condition*—one of few recent books to draw an explicit connection between health, environment, and the responsibility of physicians (Chivian, McCally, Hu, et al. 1993).

Environmental concern is also growing in bioethics. Ironically, the word *bioethics* originated in an effort to join medical and environmental ethics. Van Rensselaer Potter sought to integrate biology and the humanities, with the goal of "long-term acceptable survival of the human species." Shortly after the publication of Potter's two articles and book, in which he coined the neologism *bioethics* to join environmental and medical concerns (Potter 1971), André Hellegers and others incorporated the term into the name of the Institute for Human Reproduction and Bioethics at Georgetown University. Although Hellegers intended a more global approach to bioethics, concerns for "acceptable survival" and Aldo Leopold's land ethic fell into the background of concerns over clinical technologies and patient care (Reich 1995).

As resilient and vital as bioethics has been over the four-decade course of its development, issues of global survival and responsibility have been largely absent from its discussions. Even the bioethics books published in the last several years— some with titles referring to "critical issues for the twenty-first century"—seldom mention the broader environmental context within which medicine and ethics do their work. Bioethics risks irrelevance if it continues to ignore these issues.

The tide may be changing. Warren Reich's comprehensive second edition of the *Encyclopedia of Bioethics* includes entries on population, pollution, agriculture, environmental health, and environmental ethics. The number of articles in the bioethics literature related to environment and health, or more broadly, to nature, is small but growing. Daniel Callahan's work has consistently attended to issues of sustainability and limits in medicine, and his *False Hopes* (1998) develops the concept of sustainable medicine in detail. Some topics of central interest in bioethics involve significant global environmental issues; for example, equity in distribution of health-care resources, international research ethics, and genetic engineering. This and similar work is beginning to provide a basis for integrative work in environmental bioethics.

The environmental situation is unfolding even as we write. Still, environmental decline has been an increasingly well-recognized part of our social and material reality for many decades. Bioethics faces the challenge of coming to terms with this reality.

Humans have the power to generate meaning and structure in the face of chaos. Although the world faces a serious problem, changing our cultures could foster a rapid evolution of the material nature of our lives. As a significant element of culture, ethics has an important role to play in making this change, and thus in helping mitigate and remedy the global ecological crisis. Among other things, we can change our modes of production and how we practice health care. It may even be possible, if we take proper advantage of this moral opportunity, actually to improve the sense of meaningfulness of our lives, increase happiness, build community, and begin to maintain an adequate, sustainable global level of human healthiness.

2

Linking Health and Environmental Change

As the condition of the natural environment deteriorates, humankind faces an increasingly intractable public health crisis. At present, up to one-third of the global burden of disease, measured in terms of disability-adjusted life years (DALYs), is related to environmental factors such as poor nutrition, contaminated water, indoor smoke, vector-borne disease, and unhygienic living conditions (Murray and Lopez 1996; United Nations Environment Programme 2002, 306). Children suffer a disproportionate share of the disease and death associated with the environment, and account for two-thirds of the total environmental disease burden (United Nations Environment Programme 2002, 307). The World Health Organization estimates that environmental hazards kill some three million children under the age of five each year (United Nations Environment Programme 2002, 307). Global public health will probably get worse before it gets better: advancing at a rapid pace, environmental decline is adding to the difficulties of dealing with preventable environmental health problems related to nutrition, water, and hygiene. More unsettling still is the emergence, over the past several decades, of a host of "modern" environmental problems—climate change, ozone depletion, acid rain, toxic pollution, loss of biodiversity—that exacerbate existing environmental health problems and add unique health threats.

In this chapter we describe the major environmental challenges, both old and new, to human health. There may be some temptation, for those reading this from comfortable chairs in Boston, Omaha, or San Francisco, to feel a rather remote concern, to sympathize with the plight of the developing world but to remain unconvinced that environmental decline is relevant to patients, health-care professionals, and bioethicists in the First World. But the public health crisis is advancing among the world's relatively well-off populations as well, and the state of the global environment is critical for everyone's health.

What Is the Evidence?

The evolution of apprehension over environmental deterioration has been recorded in snapshots by the changing concerns of the United Nations decadal summit conferences on the environment. The first, convened in Stockholm 1972, signaled the emergence of concern at an international level about the state of the natural environment. The Stockholm conference focused on the release of chemical contaminants into local environments. Rachel Carson's *Silent Spring*, published in 1962, had alerted the world to the vast losses of local wildlife from the expanding use of pesticides (Carson 1962). Several serious toxic episodes had occurred, including the London air pollution disaster of 1952 and the mercury poisoning in Minimata, Japan, in 1956, and the nuclear devastation of Hiroshima and Nagasaki in 1945.

Twenty years later, at the 1992 U.N. Conference on Environment and Development in Rio de Janeiro, a new set of concerns led the agenda. Climate change represented the new shape of things. The problems were global. Without major social, technological, and economic changes, they would be difficult or impossible to solve, and they involved large-scale disruptions in feedback loops tying the earth's biosphere to the geophysical cycles that sustain life. With energy and optimism, the 1992 summit adopted a detailed set of objectives for sustainable development entitled *Agenda 21* that outlined plans and measures against which progress in resolving problems could be measured.

Nineteen-ninety-two was also the year that the Union of Concerned Scientists, on behalf of 1,600 scientists, including a majority of living Nobel laureates, issued the *World Scientists' Warning to Humanity*. Bleak and uncompromising, it outlined the destructive pressures of human activities on the atmosphere, water resources, oceans, soil, forests, and living species:

We, the undersigned senior members of the world's scientific community, hereby warn humanity of what lies ahead. A great change in our stewardship of the earth and the life of it is required, if vast human misery is to be avoided and our global home on this planet is not to be irretrievably mutilated.

(Union of Concerned Scientists, 1992)

In August of 2002, world leaders met in Johannesburg, South Africa, for the United Nations Conference on Sustainable Development. U.N. Secretary-General Kofi Annan identified five key areas for attention during the summit: water and sanitation, energy, health, agriculture, and biodiversity. The agenda reflects an emerging appreciation of the complex relationship between environmental stability and human health. It is increasingly clear that the world cannot achieve sustainable development without actively promoting human health and, at the same time, working to slow environmental degradation.

The decade from the 1992 summit to Johannesburg in 2002 showed mounting evidence of rapid environmental decline. All regions of the globe have directly experienced the effects of this decline by way of drought, flooding, fires, or epidemic disease. The global response has been excruciatingly slow. Few of the programs outlined in *Agenda 21* have been fully implemented, few of its goals have been achieved, and the health prospects of the majority of the world's population have generally become *less* secure.

The quality of environmental reporting has been refined over the past three decades. International scientific organizations have devoted significant effort to finding better, more comprehensive ways to monitor environmental trends, such as geographical information systems, remote sensing, and computer modeling. Also, data from individual nations is being more effectively collated into global data sets, allowing meaningful comparisons and global summaries. Cause-and-effect linkages are clearer. So are the complex interactions between humans and nature. Although much remains unknown or uncertain, a relatively clear picture of earth's condition is emerging from the available data.

Three Reports

Within the last few years, several large international reports on ecosystem health have added volumes of detailed information to our knowledge of the world's environmental situation (see note 1). The *Living Planet Report*, published by the World Wildlife Fund, addresses the question, "How fast is nature disappearing from the earth?" The report uses a broad range of global and national data to create a Living Planet Index (LPI) as an indicator of the overall state of the earth's natural systems. The LPI measures "natural wealth"—the area of natural forest cover around the world, and the populations of freshwater and marine species. According to the *2002 Living Planet Report*, the LPI declined overall by 37% between 1970 and 2000 (World Wildlife Fund 2002, 3).

People and Ecosystems: The Fraying Web of Life was published jointly by the United Nations Development Programme, the United Nations Environment Programme, the World Bank, and the World Resources Institute (United Nations Development Programme et al. 2000). The report presents the results of the Pilot Analysis of Global Ecosystems (PAGE) undertaken in 1999. PAGE was a collaborative effort to bring together available data on several key environmental indicators: agroecosystems and forest, freshwater, grassland, and coastal ecosystems. It gauges the condition of ecosystems by examining the services they currently provide to humans (water, food, biodiversity, carbon storage, etc.) and their capacity to continue providing these services in the future. This report identifies the major gaps and shortcomings in available global and regional data on eco-systems, and suggests where future research will be most crucial.

The Global Environment Outlook (GEO) project of the United Nations Envi-ronment Programme, initiated in 1995 in response to the global reporting require-ments of *Agenda 21*, provides comprehensive assessments on the state of the environment and directs change by building regional and international consensus on priority issues. The most recent of these GEO reports—*Global Environmental Outlook 3 (GEO-3): Past, Present and Future Perspectives*—was published in 2002, timed to contribute to the World Summit on Sustainable Development (United Nations Environment Programme 2002). GEO-3 is unique in giving cen-tral place to the notion of human vulnerability to environmental change—not only the profound impact of environmental decline on human health, but the complex synergies between poverty and environmental decline.

These three reports offer cautious, sober accounts of the state of our natural world. They leave no doubt that worldwide environmental decline is real and serious.

Water Scarcity

As we can see in photographs from outer space, the earth's surface is 80% water, making water scarcity seem an odd concern. But after accounting for the salt water of the oceans and water trapped as ice and snow, the water available for human use makes up only a tiny percent of this vast abundance, amounting proportion-ately to about a teaspoonful in a bathtub. This fraction of a percent of available water is often difficult to tap and easily polluted. "The trouble with water—and there *is* trouble with water—is that they're not making any more of it" (De Villiers 2000, 12). We have the same amount of water now as in prehistoric times.

Ground water is getting scarce. Aquifers are difficult to protect from pollution and slow to recover from it, whether it is runoff from pesticides, fertilizers, and cattle yards, or from the leaching of other toxic chemicals. In the United States, for instance, there are an estimated 10,000 underground gasoline tanks with the potential to leak into aquifers. Coastal aquifers, as they are drawn down, fill with salt water. And while rivers and lakes can recover from pollution over time and can restore lost reserves, aquifers are slower to regenerate—particularly when the land on top of them subsides. Both the Ogallala aquifer, which underlies 170,000 square miles of the Great Plains and is the largest U.S. water source, and the Nubian aquifer, which underlies a large section of Africa, are being used up much more quickly than they can replenish.

Most, if not all, of the fresh water on the planet is to some degree contaminated, most obviously in urban and industrial areas. Yet even the far reaches of the sea are subject to fallout from the atmosphere and from wide dispersal of oil, garbage, chemicals, and human sewage. Even on the remotest beaches, plastic bags and tampon applicators and other signs of distant human activities wash ashore. Oceans, streams, lakes, deltas, wetlands, estuaries, aquifers—none remain untouched.

Rivers and lakes are affected by point and nonpoint sources of pollution. *Point* sources—where pollution is discharged at a particular site—include factories and sewage pipes, and are somewhat easier to monitor than *nonpoint* sources such as runoff from feedlots and farmlands. Oceans are perhaps our most polluted waters, since they have served for many years as a global dumping ground for the daily garbage from boats, for millions of tons of dredge spoils, and for an endless supply of raw human and animal sewage.

Inadequate supplies of water pose major problems for public health, evidenced in the staggering statistics of suffering and death related to water worldwide. Over a billion people lack access to clean drinking water, and 31 countries are water-scarce. Groups gathered at a recent international symposium on water predicted that by 2025 two-thirds of the world's population will be living with water shortages or absolute water scarcity (Institute for Food and Development Policy 2001, 1). A recent international report on the health of children estimated that water- and food-borne diarrhoeal diseases claim the lives of at least two million children each year and "have killed more children in the last ten years than all people lost to armed conflict since World War II" (United Nations Environment Programme, United Nations Children's Fund, and World Health Organization 2002, 47).

Soil and Food Production

Although dirt is unlimited in supply, the kind that produces food is actually quite scarce. Each year, millions of tons of topsoil are blown or washed away. As a soil scientist quipped, "The problem is that people treat soil like dirt." The largest factors driving land degradation are agriculture, especially livestock production, and the conversion of forests to croplands. Land suffers from salinization and waterlogging caused by excessive irrigation, an overload of pesticides and fertilizers, and compaction by the use of heavy farming machinery. Urban development, roads, malls, and the like cover fertile soil with asphalt and cement. By far the commonest form of degradation is erosion, where wind and water carry away nutrient-rich topsoil—exposed by logging and careless farming, or development.

This large-scale loss of fertile agricultural potential bodes ill for the world's rapidly expanding and already hungry population. Although it is well established that the starvation and malnutrition suffered by segments of the world's population are not primarily a consequence of global food shortages but rather of maldistribution, political instability, and geographic bad luck, environmental degradation is likely to strike first at the food supply of already threatened populations. And even if absolute scarcity of food does not presently constitute the immediate cause of famines, it is strengthening as an underlying factor.

Food production has increased dramatically in the last half century, and has so far kept pace with population growth. But the ability of ecosystems to continue producing enough food is less certain. High food production has been achieved, in part, by converting large areas of land to managed agroecosystems. Fertilizers, particularly nitrogen, have allowed farmers to dramatically increase crop yields. But the state of the world's agroecosystems is declining. According to a World Resources report, about two-thirds of agricultural land has been degraded in the past fifty years, placing considerable constraints on future productivity (United Nations Development Programme et al. 2000, 10). Not only land degradation, but many other global environmental trends directly threaten agricultural production. For example, climate change will probably disrupt rainfall patterns, while increased ultraviolet-B (UV-B) radiation will damage plants by disrupting photosynthesis.

Research by the United States Department of Agriculture suggests that, although the world witnessed a significant increase in food production in the 1950s to 1990, this trend has leveled off. Although the annual increase in world grain yield before 1990 averaged 2.1% per year, the annual rate of increase for the 1990s was only 1.2%, and there is reason to be concerned about the capacity of the world to maintain even this rate of increase during the next decades (Brown 2001, 51). Even those who are optimistic about agriculture's ability to accommodate expected population growth note that this can only be accomplished by substantial improvements and new investments in agricultural policies and techniques. Increased damage to environmental resources must be expected (Bongaarts 1996, 499).

The future of fish production—a vital source of food for many of the world's people—is also uncertain. Coastal ecosystems are among the most stressed, and stocks of the world's most important fish are depleted or overharvested (United Nations Development Programme et al. 2000, 12). The increasing use of aquaculture, and the decline of natural fish stocks, will be particularly hard on those who depend on subsistence fishing.

Vaclav Smil has addressed the question of how we might best feed the ten billion people who will probably inhabit the earth by 2050 (Smil 2000). He argues vigorously for a rapid and humane transition to a stabilized population and for significant changes in how we farm and eat. There are vast disparities in average grain consumption, based not only on the amount of food eaten, but on the percentage of grain used to produce meat and dairy products. For example, the average consumption of grain per capita in North America is about 700 kg per year; in Africa it is just over 200 kg (World Wildlife Fund 1999, 10). About a third of the global grain harvest is fed to animals—which is why Smil and others strongly recommend a shift toward mainly vegetarian diets. Smil notes:

[E]ven today's six billion people could not be fed if North America's current average per capita food supply (of which about 40 percent is wasted!) were to become the global norm in a world that would be using much higher agricultural inputs with no better efficiencies than we do today.

(Smil 2000, ix)

Climate Change

Earth maintains a relatively constant temperature by the complex interactions of atmospheric gases, solar heat, and various terrestrial and aquatic processes. Earth absorbs radiation from the sun, and then redistributes some of this energy back into space in longer, thermal wavelengths. Some of this radiation is taken up by a layer of "greenhouse gases" in the atmosphere and re-radiated back to earth, warming its surface. The greater the concentration of greenhouse gases, the more effectively heat is trapped and re-radiated back to earth. In 1896, Svante August Arrhenius, a Swedish chemist, theorized that the carbon dioxide released by burning fossil fuels would add to the accumulation of greenhouse gases and would have a warming effect on earth's atmosphere.

His theory has been borne out. Over the past century, a steadily and rapidly increasing concentration of greenhouse gases has caused an increase in the amount of heat retained by earth's atmosphere. A 2001 report by the Intergovernmental Panel on Climate Change (IPCC), representing a consensus of the world's leading atmospheric scientists, concludes that global average temperature has increased since 1861. It is "very likely" that the 1990s were the warmest decade and 1998 the warmest year in the instrumental record (since 1861) (IPCC 2001b, 2). Observations collected over the last century suggest that average land surface temperature has risen 0.45–0.6°C (0.8–1.0°F) in the last century. Precipitation has increased by about 0.5–1% on average globally, and the sea level has risen worldwide approximately 15–20cm (6–8 inches) in the last century (Environmental Protection Agency 2002).

Rapidly mounting observational evidence indicates that ecosystems have already been affected. Examples of observed changes include shrinking glaciers, thawing permafrost, later freezing and earlier breakup of ice on rivers and lakes, lengthening of mid- to high-latitude growing seasons, poleward and altitudinal shifting of plant and animal ranges, declining plant and animal populations, and earlier tree flowering, insect emergence, and bird egg-laying (IPCC 2001a, 11).

Over the next century, climate model predictions project an increase in globally averaged surface temperature of between 1.4°C and 5.8°C (IPCC 2001a, 5). The effects of these changes on both a global and regional scale are unknown, although refined scientific models have been developed to predict effects on various aspects of earth's ecosystems, such as significant slowing of the ocean circulation that transports water to the North Atlantic, and large reductions in the Greenland and west Antarctic ice sheets. Global warming may be accelerated by carbon cycle feedbacks in the terrestrial biosphere, by releases of terrestrial carbon from permafrost regions, and by releases of methane from hydrates in the coastal sediments.

Changes in global atmospheric patterns are expected to affect human health in many ways. The most direct impact would be exposure to heat or cold. Events like the summer heat wave of 1995 in Chicago, which caused numerous deaths in the city, will probably become more frequent. Scientists have created complex mathematical models for estimating the potential effects of climate change on vector-borne diseases. These models project increases in the worldwide transmission of malaria, dengue fever, and cholera, and a decrease in schistosomiasis. Heavy rains might cause outbreaks of cryptosporidiosis; unusual cycles of drought and rain might be linked to outbreaks of hantavirus (Haines, McMichael, and Epstein 2000, 732). Epidemiologists are exploring whether the recent resurgence of infectious diseases such as tuberculosis and malaria as well as the appearance of newly recognized viruses such as marburg and ebola might be related to climate warming (Garrett 1994). The expected flooding and denudation resulting from the sea level rise is likely to cause extensive harm to human health through food deprivation, pollution, relocation, and the spread of diseases (Haines, McMichael, and Epstein 2000, 732–733).

In 1992, reacting to scientific concern about increasing concentrations of greenhouse gases, most nations of the world signed the United Nations Framework Convention on Climate Change. The 1992 treaty included a voluntary, non-binding pledge that the major industrialized nations would reduce greenhouse emissions to 1990 levels by the year 2000. Over the next few years, it became clear that major greenhouse producers such as the United States and Japan would not meet voluntary targets; at the same time, scientific concern about the effects of warming—which by now had been definitively linked to human activities—intensified. In 1995, negotiations began on a protocol to establish legally binding limitations or reductions on greenhouse emissions.

The Kyoto Protocol was completed in 1997. The protocol aims for a reduction of overall emissions of six key greenhouse gases (carbon dioxide, methane, nitrous oxide, hydrofluorocarbons, perfluorocarbons, and sulphur hexafluoride) by an average of 5.2% below 1990 levels during the commitment period of 2008 to 2012. The United States would have been obligated to a 7% cumulative reduction. The Protocol took effect in 2002 when it was ratified by 55% of the nations emitting at least 55% of the greenhouse gases. The United States, which accounts for about 25% of global emissions, with 4% of the world's population, signed the Protocol in 1998, but President Bush withdrew the United States from the treaty in March of 2001.

Reservations about the Kyoto Protocol arise from various sources. Some rightly point out that much deeper reductions in carbon output—reductions on the order of two-thirds according to one study (Kauppi 1995)—will be needed to affect the climate significantly. But climate activists see the Protocol as a first step and a mechanism by which deeper cuts can be made and wider participation obtained. Others wonder whether the expense of societal change is worth the good to be sought (Lomborg 2001). Environmentalists generally hold the economic criticism to be shortsighted.

Stratospheric Ozone Depletion

Hovering in the stratosphere between 12 and 30 miles above the earth, a layer of ozone molecules acts as life's sunscreen, allowing only a fraction of the sun's ultraviolet radiation to reach the surface of the planet. Without the ozone layer, the sun's radiant energy would make earth as uninhabitable as Mars. In 1974, chemists Sherwood Rowland and Mario Molina published a paper suggesting that stratospheric ozone might be destroyed by manmade substances such as the chlorofluorocarbons (CFCs) found in refrigerators, air conditioners, and cans of hairspray. The first major "hole" in the ozone layer was discovered in the 1980s over Antarctica. Since then, various levels of depletion have been recorded over both the northern and southern hemispheres (de Gruijl and van der Leun 2000, 851).

Stratospheric ozone depletion results in increased levels of solar radiation reaching the earth's surface and the top layers of the ocean. The long-term effects on humans and ecosystems are still somewhat uncertain. Destruction of crops is an obvious concern, though scientists' worries focus on more extensive effects on all plant life. For instance, ocean phytoplankton, which forms a basic link in the earth's food chain, is highly vulnerable to UV-B damage and has experienced a marked decline in recent years.

Increased radiation has had adverse health consequences for humans, marked particularly by a dramatic upsurge in skin cancers—squamous cell carcinomas, basal cell carcinomas, and cutaneous malignant melanomas. Other health effects are less well studied. Increased UV-B radiation may be linked to cataracts and retinal degeneration, and has been shown to suppress the immune system (de Gruijl and van der Leun 2000, 852–4).

The ozone situation has some hopeful aspects. The Montreal Protocol, one of the most effective international efforts to control ecological deterioration, has been widely accepted by nations, which have agreed to reduce production of ozone-depleting CFCs. In the mid-1990s, worldwide emissions dropped to levels about 40 percent below those of 1986—less than amounts permitted under the Montreal Protocol. The total combined abundance of ozone depleting substances in the lower atmosphere is now declining, after reaching its peak in 1994.

Estimating the extent of damage is made difficult by the ten-year time lag between the release of CFCs and their migration to the middle stratosphere. For example, the health effects of past emissions—particularly skin cancers and eye damage—may not yet be in evidence. There are further complexities. Ozone depletion interacts with several other global trends, such as climate change and air pollution. The loss of stratospheric ozone has caused a cooling of the lower stratosphere, and may have offset as much as 30 percent of the warming effect of other greenhouse gases. On the other hand, the effects of ozone depletion on fish and aquatic plants may have been heightened because decreased organic carbon levels in lakes—the result of acid rain—allow UV-B radiation to penetrate more deeply into surface waters (United Nations Environment Programme 2000).

Nitrogen Loading

The availability and transfer of certain chemical elements in the environment are key factors affecting life on earth. Biogeochemical cycles—nutrients moving among rock, air, soil, water, and living organisms—regulate the global chemical balance. A number of the most pressing environmental concerns relate to human-induced imbalances in these cycles—we have already looked at the ozone layer and at greenhouse gases. Another important chemical cycle being altered by human activities is the nitrogen cycle. Concern about nitrogen loading is relatively new in environmental circles, and is quickly becoming a focus of attention. Nitrogen, a constituent of all plant and animal tissues, occurs in proteins and nucleic acid, and forms nearly 80% of the atmosphere by volume. Although widely present in the atmosphere, nitrogen must be fixed by nitrogen-absorbing microorganisms in the soil and water and by nitrogen-fixing plants before it is available for use. Human activities have permanently altered the distribution of nitrogen on earth and made huge quantities of nitrogen available for uptake by plants (Smil 1991; Vitousek 1994). We are literally over-fertilizing the earth.

The most important source of anthropogenic (human-made) nitrogen is inorganic nitrogen fertilizer. Farmers have long known that a shortage of nitrogen can limit biological productivity, and have traditionally used crop rotations (growing legumes, which are good nitrogen-fixers) and nitrogen-rich animal waste to boost productivity. Early in the twentieth century, a process was developed to synthesize ammonia, creating an artificial nitrogen fertilizer. Nitrogen fertilizer has been a powerful tool in allowing food production to keep pace with population growth during this century (Smil 1997). But the introduction of massive quantities of nitrogen into soils and waters has a number of negative consequences for the environment and human health.

Researchers have noted a large rise in nitrogen levels in drinking water supplies, particularly in agricultural areas. Indeed, nitrate pollution is considered one of the most serious water quality problems globally. High nitrate levels have been linked to cancers (Smil 1997, 79) and to methaemoglobineamia or "blue baby syndrome" (United Nations Environment Program, United Nations Children's Fund, World Health Organization 2002, 61). Nitric oxide is a precursor of ground-level ozone, a component of smog, dangerous to human health and crop productivity. It can be transformed into nitric acid, which washes out of the atmosphere as acid rain. Rising levels of nitrogen have led to increased algal and plant growth, and also to *eutrophication* of lakes and rivers—where rapid growth of algae and cyanobacteria in the water deprives other species of oxygen. Some research suggests that damage to coastal ecosystems and declines in fish stocks can be blamed on the "nutrient enrichment" of too much nitrogen. The incidence of red or brown tides—large algal blooms that damage ocean life—has also been related to nitrogen loading. Elevated nitrogen levels can have a wide variety of impacts on land ecosystems, such as increased leaching of potassium and calcium (which regulate soil acidity), and a reduction in biodiversity (by enhancing the growth of some plants while hindering the growth of others).

Unlike carbon loading in the atmosphere, which has economically and technically feasible solutions, there is no way to decrease our reliance on nitrogen fertilizers without lowering food production (Smil 1997). Stabilization of population growth may then be a key response. Also, a large-scale adoption of a vegetarian diet could keep nitrogen use in check, since feeding grain to humans is far more direct and efficient than feeding grain to cattle (Smil 1997; Smil 2000). Finally, farmers can learn to be far more efficient in their use of fertilizers; for example, monitoring the level of useable nitrogen in soil and only applying fertilizer when needed (Smil 1997).

Toxic Chemicals

One of the most serious environmental health problems in the world is air pollution. Over a billion people breathe unhealthy air, and some five percent of the global burden of disease is attributable to air pollution, second only to the toll associated with unclean water (United Nations Environment Programme 2002, 307). In developing countries, indoor air pollution from burning biomass and fossil fuel is a major cause of illness, particularly acute respiratory infection. Other health problems associated with poor indoor air quality include chronic respiratory diseases such as lung cancer and bronchitis. There is also increasing evidence that air quality affects the unborn child: stillbirths and low birth weight are associated with exposure to air pollutants during pregnancy (United Nations Environment Programme, United Nations Children's Fund, World Health Organization 2002, 72). Outdoor air pollution is equally serious. People living in cities are exposed to a vast number of toxins, including carbon monoxide, nitrogen oxide, sulphur dioxide, lead, suspended particulates, dioxins, and volatile organic compounds. Studied health effects of poor outdoor air quality include asthma, emphysema, bronchitis, lung cancer, and impaired fetal growth and infant development (United Nations Environment Programme, United Nations Children's Fund, World Health Organization 2002, 69–72).

Toxic exposures also occur from water, particularly drinking water, which might, for example, contain nitrates from pesticide runoff or heavy metals leached into groundwater from a landfill. Arsenic, which occurs naturally in ground water, also poses a serious health threat in some areas of the world.

Lead exposure in children has been a particularly vexing problem in the United States. Although lead exposure has been greatly reduced, pockets of the population, primarily the poor, continue to be exposed to high levels of lead in deteriorating household paint, and large numbers of people are exposed to lead in outdoor air pollution and in food. Lead exposure has been linked, among other things, to impaired neurobehavioral development in children (Brooks et al. 1995, 385). Mercury has been another heavy metal of particular concern, primarily because of several serious large-scale exposures, including the epidemic in Japan known as Minimata disease, where a large number of the villagers living in Minimata Bay developed a strange and debilitating neurological disease after eating mercury-laced fish. The largest source of mercury exposure for humans has been fish, which rapidly absorb methylmercury from polluted aquatic environments. Human absorption of methylmercury into the bloodstream and finally the tissues is highly efficient. Health effects include bilateral constriction of vision, ataxia, tremors, dementia, and congenital neurological deformities (Brooks et al. 1995, 132).

Another group of chemicals called persistent organic pollutants (POPs) has been generating increasing concern. These chemicals include polychlorinated biphenyls (PCBs), pesticides such as aldrin, chlordane, DDT, dieldrin, and heptachlor, and industrial byproducts such as dioxins. POPs are fat-soluble, accumulate in fatty tissues of animals, and concentrate as they move up the food chain, where, because they are chemically stable, they can persist over long periods of time. DDT, for example, is a highly persistent insecticide: traces of DDT have been found all over the world, even in the fatty tissues of Antarctic penguins (Steingraber 1998; Thornton 2000). Although DDT is no longer manufactured in the United States, it is still produced in several foreign countries. Despite its dangers, DDT is considered one of the most effective means to control malaria.

Concern about POPs has intensified with the emergence of scientific research suggesting that certain POPs appear to mimic hormones. These so-called endocrine disruptors or *environmental estrogens* may play a role in a range of human and environmental health problems, particularly related to reproduction and development.

Endocrine disruptors have long been a source of concern to wildlife biologists, who reported various abnormalities in wildlife exposed to these chemicals: feminization of males, birth defects, altered sex ratios, decreased sperm density, breast cancer, and testicular cancer (Solomon and Schettler 2000, 1472). Already, a number of amphibian and bird species have shown declines that researchers believe are related to chemical exposure (Colborn, Dumanoski, and Myers 1996). Recent research also suggests that estrogenic compounds may disrupt nitrogen fixation—the process by which leguminous plants in symbiotic relationship with nitrogen-fixing bacteria make nitrogen available for use by living organisms (Fox et al. 2001).

The effects of POPs and environmental estrogens on humans is still uncertain, but it is extremely unlikely that these classes of chemicals, with so many potent effects on so many species, would somehow leave humans untouched. Epidemiological studies on occupational exposures to certain pesticides and industrial chemicals have shown diminished sperm quality and quantity, impaired sexual function, increased testicular cancer, and adverse effects on offspring such as hypospadias and cryptorchidism (Solomon and Schettler 2000, 1472). Although population-based studies are limited, as is the scientific understanding of gene–environment interactions, researchers worry that as epidemiologic data and scientific understanding improve—and when these chemicals have been under scrutiny long enough that the time-lag between exposure and effect can be integrated into the research—we may see that there has already been a profound impact on human health. Some of the health effects we may see include increases in certain cancers (particularly those of the reproductive organs), infertility, birth defects, and thyroid disruption.

Biodiversity

Estimating rates of species loss is difficult, since there is no well-established baseline count of the numbers of species that actually exist. Biologists estimate that between five and thirty million species of plants, animals, and microorganisms currently exist on earth. The rate of species loss may be anywhere between 2000 and 30,000 species each year, a pace that is most likely accelerating. Two kinds of biodiversity, each equally important to the survival of life on earth, are at risk: diversity of species, and genetic variability among individuals of a particular species. The rapid loss of species threatens ecosystem stability because of the interdependencies that link species together. Reduction in numbers within a species can lead to the loss of races and varieties. When a species is dramatically reduced in numbers and loses genetic sub-units, it is less resilient, less able to adapt to changes, and thus more vulnerable to events such as climate change, disease, or loss of habitat. Moreover, the dominance of human habitats is reducing the ability of many species to migrate in response to global climate change (Walther et al. 2002).

Because measuring species loss is so inexact, some analyses of biodiversity focus instead on the state of natural ecosystems, which provides a rough picture of how species are faring. The *Living Planet Report* (LPR)—whose driving concern is biodiversity—brings together the available data on three major indicators of ecosystem health: the area of natural forest cover around the world, populations of freshwater species, and populations of marine species.

The world's forest ecosystems have declined significantly. According to the Living Planet Index, natural forest cover was reduced by 10% between 1970 and 1995: equivalent to the loss, every year, of an area larger than Florida or Bangladesh (World Wildlife Fund 1999, 4). Populations of species living in forest ecosystems have declined an estimated 15% between 1970 and 2000 (World Wildlife Fund 2002, 3).

Even in areas such as North America and Europe, where forest cover has remained constant, the health of forests has suffered. Replacement of old-growth forest with single-species tree plantations, and the fragmentation of forests into areas too small to support populations of certain species, have led to the decline or loss of a number of plants, animals, and insects.

Loss, degradation, and pollution of the earth's forests is likely to affect humans through increasing scarcity of wood-based resources (wood is widely used throughout the world for cooking), loss of potential biological knowledge, and especially, broad and complex reverberations within earth's ecosystems. Changes in forest cover will affect moisture patterns, which will in turn lead to changes in soil cover, particularly through the loss of topsoil to erosion and wind. Forested watersheds recharge streams, springs, and aquifers. Trees prevent soil erosion and absorb noise and pollution. Forests contribute medicinal drugs: the World Health Organization estimates that 80% of the world's population relies on traditional plant-based medicines. Plant species also provide a rich source for pharmaceutical research (Baker et al. 1995; Soejarto 1996). Over half of the world's plant species are found in tropical forests.

To measure the health of freshwater ecosystems, the LPR tracked the population trends of 102 freshwater vertebrate species, including mammals, birds, amphibians, and fish. Since 1970, freshwater species have, on average, declined by about 45% (World Wildlife Fund 1999, 6). Already one-fifth of the world's freshwater fish are either endangered or extinct. Scientists have been particularly alarmed by the decline in amphibian species, many of which live in protected habitats. Research has suggested a link to pollution (e.g., such POPs as dioxin) and to increased ultraviolet radiation. But the loss of these species is still largely unexplained (World Wildlife Fund 1999, 6).

The LPR also tracks the average change in population of 102 species of marine fish, reptiles, birds, and mammals. Between 1970 and 1995, populations have declined by about 35% (World Wildlife Fund 1999, 8). The causes of species loss in marine environments include loss of habitat, pollution, and overharvesting. The loss of wetlands, mangroves, and sea grasses has meant that coastal areas have lost some capacity to filter pollutants, thereby increasing the frequency of harmful algae blooms and hypoxia. Marine environments are also contaminated by oil spills. The *Exxon Valdez* spill seemed like an unusually disastrous event because of the media attention; yet the 11-million-gallon spill was relatively small and not out of the ordinary (240 million gallons were spilled during the 1991 Persian Gulf war, and 140 million gallons during a 1979–1980 spill in the Gulf of Mexico). Chronic small spills and leakage from ocean-based pumping operations may be even more damaging to ecosystems than large but isolated spills, since ecosystems have a more difficult time recovering from repeated assaults (Burger 1997). Sometimes the loss of species can occur for reasons one might not anticipate. For instance, marine biologists have noted a link between whaling and the slow extinction of some deep-sea creatures (species we are just now beginning to discover). When they sink to the bottom of the ocean, whale skeletons become homes to whole communities of deep-sea life that thrive there and nowhere else. Intensive whaling has reduced the number of skeletons on the sea floor, making life hard for those creatures relying on this curious habitat (Butman, Carlton, and Palumbi 1995).

The relevance of biodiversity to medicine is quite direct: many pharmaceuticals are developed or derived from organisms found in nature, such as digitalis from foxglove and aspirin from willow bark. As Eric Chivian notes, organisms from the tropical rain forests "have given us d-tubocururine (from the chondodendron vine), quinine and quinidine (from the cinchona tree), vinblastine and vincristine (from the rosy periwinkle plant), and erythromycin, neomycin, and amphotericin (from soil microbes)" (Chivian 2001, 66). Vast numbers of species remain unstudied, so with tropical forests under particular strain, losses of great pharmaceutical potential can be expected.

Biodiversity also has much broader, though perhaps less obvious, importance for human well-being. Ecosystems provide a number of "services" we rely on: filtering pollutants from water, forming soil, pollinating plants, providing food and fuel, and regulating the biogeochemical cycles of oxygen, carbon, and nitrogen in the atmosphere (see note 2). When we stress and destabilize ecosystems, we decrease their capacity to perform these services—services we take for granted when all is working well. But we can neither do without them nor easily replace them technologically.

Unpredictability and Natural Disasters

Floods, volcanoes, earthquakes, storm surges, hurricanes, tornados, droughts, and landslides have always been a part of the human story. Yet the gods seem to be getting angrier these days, hurling down one catastrophe after another. In 1998, at least 10,000 lives were lost when Hurricane Mitch slammed into Central America; another thousand lost their lives in a cyclone in Gujarat, India in 1998. Extensive forests burned in Indonesia, affecting about 70 million people there and in neighboring countries, and causing an estimated $9.3 billion in damage. In 1999, landslides in Venezuela claimed another 30,000 lives and caused untold economic damage. In the *World Disasters Report 2002*, the International Federation of Red Cross and Red Crescent Societies estimated that the number of people affected by disasters in the 1990s totaled nearly two billion altogether, a significant increase compared to the 700 million in the decade of the 1970s (Walter 2002, Chap. 8). During the decade of the 1990s, natural disasters caused over $608 billion in economic damage, "more than in the previous four decades combined" (Abramovitz 2001, 123).

Several trends have increased the frequency and seriousness of natural disasters. Although the number of geophysical disasters such as earthquakes has remained steady, their impact on humans has been amplified. Human settlements are denser, and more people now live along coastlines and seismic fault lines. Because ecosystems are stressed, they are less resilient when hit by a natural event such as drought, fire, or heavy rain, paving the way for an "event" to become a disaster. The number of hydro-meteorological disasters has more than doubled in the past five years. Various explanations are given for the increase: floods are worse when forests are cleared; overgrazing can intensify the effects of drought. Global warming, since it raises the energy levels of the atmosphere, makes weather patterns more erratic and more extreme. A rising sea level will put even more people at risk of flooding. Population growth has also pushed people to settle in areas that are sensitive to disaster: the urban rich, in trying to sequester themselves, perch their houses on cliffs and mountainsides; the poor, in trying to survive, settle on the only lands available, those subject to floods or drought.

Natural disasters are highly unpredictable, and the rapidly shifting scale and unexpected interactions of environmental processes are likely to pass as-yet-unperceived thresholds. As Norman Myers warns, "When one problem combines with another problem, the outcome may be not a double problem but a super problem" (1995, 360).

Conclusion

As Boyden and Dovers note, "Ominous changes in the biosphere are already evident at regional and global levels" (Boyden and Dovers 1992, 67). These environmental changes and consequent health problems are not easily remedied (see note 3). Their depth and extent this century will significantly affect the goals and the nature of health care everywhere on the planet. Poor health, illnesses, and injuries will probably increase, and the causes of these conditions will increasingly be global environmental conditions. Meanwhile, the resources available for health-care systems to mitigate the individual consequences of global change are likely to decline. If health care is to continue to play a significant role in our health, we will need to adapt our health practices to these new conditions.

In order to appreciate how fundamentally our conceptions of health care must change, we need to review some of the current dynamics of population and consumption that are driving ecosystem decline. This we do in the next chapter as we explore the problem of finding an ethical and balanced response to limiting population and consumption.

Notes for Chapter 2

1. Environments and Ecosystems

An *environment* is "the circumstances, objects, or conditions by which one is surrounded." An *ecosystem* is "the complex of a community of organisms and its environment functioning as an ecological unit in nature" (*Webster's Collegiate Dictionary*, 10th ed.). The earth is the home of a single biological ecosystem that embraces various regional subsystems. The term *ecosystem* connotes a global coherence and holism that environmentalists urge us to respect. *Environment* is less coherent and more ambiguous. For instance, if one were to search Medline for the "environment" of medicine, one would mostly find articles on the regulatory and economic "environment" of health care. We want to place medical services firmly in the context of earth's one great ecosystem.

2. Ecosystem Services

Ecosystem services commonly identified and studied include:

- Regulation of atmospheric chemical composition
- Regulation of climate (including global temperature, precipitation, and other biologically mediated climatic processes)
- Regulation of hydrological flows
- Mitigation of floods and droughts
- Storage and retention of water (in aquifers, watersheds, reservoirs)
- Soil formation, soil fertility, and erosion control
- Nutrient cycling (e.g., nitrogen fixation)
- Waste treatment (removal or breakdown of excess and toxic nutrients and compounds)
- Pollination and seed dispersal (which allow for reproduction of plants)
- Control of most agricultural pests
- Habitat, human and otherwise
- Support of human diversity
- Support of biodiversity and genetic resources
- The beauty and grandeur of earth's natural world
  (Adapted from Costanza et al. 1997, 254; and Daily 1997)

3. Energy Sources and Entropy

Energy flow is a key concept for appreciating the limits of the earth in an integrated way. The flow of solar energy onto the planet sets the earth's energy budget for the movement of air and water, the growth and evolution of life, and the conduct of any activity. For most of human history, humans have been dependent primarily on the energy they have been able to draw for food and work from plants and microorganisms capable of capturing sunlight. Currently, humans are operating on an energy budget many times what can be recovered on a sustainable basis from these sources. By the 1980s, Vitousek and others estimated that humans were using roughly half of the globe's net annual energy capture by these sources (Vitousek et al. 1986), and a similar estimate in 2002 finds humans using about a fifth more than earth's biological restorative capacity (Wackernagel et al. 2002).

Many of the problems we have described in this chapter involve the widespread distribution and mixing of materials at the molecular level—nitrogen, acid rain (hydrogen), environmental estrogens, heavy metals, and so on. To sequester these thinly distributed materials, to purify air and water, and then to return the air, water, and materials to usable form requires lots of energy, engineering, and social organization. Bottom line: "it is much harder to get the cream out of the coffee than to pour it in" (Leonard Rifas, personal communication, 1978).

Humans have extended their energy use mainly by harnessing fossil and nuclear fuels. In the case of fossil fuels, humans are drawing on energy banked by plants and animals over millions of years. There is a catch to using these fuels. According to well-studied laws of thermodynamics, when we use energy, it inevitably changes from more useful forms to less useful ones. This decrease in the utility of energy is sometimes termed *entropy*. When energy is used in a closed system, the entropy of that system increases—always. To overcome the increase in entropy, the world can use some of the day's input of solar energy, but that input is limited by the capacity of the earth's plants and microorganisms to transform solar energy into useful structure and energy-bearing materials.

Entropy is a kind of chaos, so using more energy inevitably causes chaos. Global warming is one of the dangerous kinds of chaos caused by high levels of energy generation and use. Carbon and other greenhouse gases in the atmosphere represent part of the entropic cost of fossil fuel use. Using additional fossil fuel to repair other environmental problems would then buy an even greater entropy problem than we now have. Nuclear fuels are even worse than fossil fuels in this regard, because the entropic effect of using nuclear energy is to create long-term waste that is violently chaotic and toxic.

Because of these limitations of fossil and nuclear fuels, and because a lot of the energy from the sun that falls on earth is not captured by plants, environmentalists are hopeful about wind and solar energy. Yet even if solar and wind energy can be harnessed safely and at low environmental cost, it will take many years and an immense investment of capital to build a system that can even begin to displace the present scale of energy expenditure. It is impossible to imagine this fundamental transition in energy technologies taking place without necessary and consequential changes in culture, modes of production, and the nature of consumption.

It is unlikely that our current high-energy societies can long endure. And the technologies and industry of high-energy societies can provide solutions neither to the world's production problems nor to the restoration of the natural world.

(Sources: Smil 1994; Price 1995, McNeill 2001, Peet 1992, Vitousek 1997; Georgescu-Roegen 1995)

3

Population and Consumption

The various stresses on earth's ecosystems described in Chapter 2 result from the combined effects of global levels of population and consumption. Population growth has been widely discussed and debated, and institutionalized approaches to limiting population growth, albeit imperfect, are in place around the globe. The moral dimensions of population growth and limitation have also been considered, though bioethics itself has remained relatively quiet on the subject in recent years.

The problems of consumption, on the other hand, have not been as widely recognized in the United States. Although many people are committing their time and ingenuity to the problems of overconsumption, institutions for change are not in place. Indeed, many of the dominant cultural institutions appear to be fundamentally committed to growth. At every level of public discourse, growth proponents attack alternative viewpoints with confidence, ideology, and propaganda (Proctor 1994). Similarly, little has been said about the ethics of consumption as it relates to human health, to health care, and to health-care ethics. In order to draw conclusions about this realm in health care, we need first to provide some background on why ethics should take very seriously the issue of limiting consumption in the First World.

Reaching the Limits of Population and Consumption

A Short History of Growth

For most of the time span humans have inhabited the planet (perhaps three million years), human population has grown slowly. By A.D. 1, the earth probably hosted 200–400 hundred million people. The count did not reach a billion until about the beginning of the nineteenth century (around the time that Jeremy Bentham wrote his utilitarian theory that the happiness of each person counts equally). During the twentieth century, the world saw a sharp acceleration in population growth. By 1930, the world had added a second billion, and by 1960, a third. It took only fifteen years more to reach four billion, and then twelve years to reach five. Although the rate of natural increase dropped after 1990, the world added another billion people between 1987 and 1998 to reach six billion. At the time of this writing, the U.S. Census Bureau population clock reads about 6.30 billion.

The fertility rate has been declining during the thirty years since it peaked in about 1970. The number of couples using family planning in less developed countries has increased from less than 10% in the 1960s to almost 60% today (Ashford et al. 2002). Still, at current levels of growth, the human population is increasing at about 75 million people per year. Despite declines in fertility, the world is committed to continued population growth for the next several decades. This growth momentum continues because the population base is very large, and the number of people at or approaching reproductive age increased in recent decades.

Population projections released by the United Nations in 2000 estimate that world population will be between 7.9 and 10.9 billion by 2050 (United Nations 2000, 5). Whether the human population peaks out at the higher or lower end of these projections depends on a number of factors. For example, if support for international family planning remains spotty, numbers may edge toward the higher end (Speidel 2000, 552). A rise in HIV infections and a decline in fertility may pull the numbers back toward mid-range.

People in the developed nations, especially those in the United States, often feel that they are exempt from population concerns, that growth is solely the concern of the developing world and that the main objective should be to limit the growth of other regions of the world. Yet at 285 million people (in round numbers, 5% of the world population), the United States is the world's third-most-populous nation and has one of the highest rates of natural increase of all industrialized nations.

Meanwhile, per capita use of the earth's resources has also been increasing. As with population growth, most of this intensification of human industrial activity has taken place in the last century. Indeed, during the last 100 years, most of the aggregate global consumption and production curves rose more sharply than population. According to J. R. McNeill, the population quadrupled while the overall global economy grew by a factor of fourteen, overall energy use grew sixteen times, carbon dioxide emissions seventeen times, industrial output forty times, and water use nine times (McNeill 2000, 360).

The Existence of Limits

According to many scientists, environmental decline is largely driven by this dynamic combination of human population growth with the burgeoning intensity and destructiveness of human consumption—a "technometabolism" that ravages the earth's resources (Goodland 1992; McNeill 2002, 16–17; Meadows, Meadows, and Randers 1992; Wackernagel et al. 2002). But, the global ecosystem is a closed biological system and therefore finite in its capacity to supply energy and materials and to serve as a sink for waste. For most of human history, territorial expansion was slow enough and technology modest enough that the biosphere was relatively safe from the harmful consequences of human activity.

Although humans have so far generally been able to continue to expand their consumption of earth's resources, the long-standing assumption that the earth has an infinite capacity to serve our needs is being displaced by a paradigm of limits. It is becoming clear that although technological innovation may increase the capacity and efficiency of production, these processes are subject to terrestrial limits set by sources of supply and access to the means of waste disposal.

If it is to function sustainably, every form of technology, whether old or new, must function within limits set by the earth. All forms of production should be traced back to their ultimate dependency on nature's resources and services. Genetic innovations in food plants such as wheat and rice must face the limits set by available water supply, nitrogen and trace minerals in the soil, and the stability and favorableness of weather. The expansion of agriculture through the heavy use of synthetic nitrogen must face the limits set by global warming and nitrogen pollution. More materials can be recovered from the industrial waste stream and recycled, but these processes also require the substantial use of limited energy resources. Entropic costs can only be bled off at a rate that the biosphere can maintain.

It appears that humans are currently straining earth's capacities to the point of fracture. Perhaps the most powerful indication that we are nearing earth's limits is the present *de facto* rapid decline in the natural world as the intensity of human activity escalates. According to several analysts, the technological subsystem has gone "beyond the limits" (Meadows, Meadows, and Randers 1992) and is reaching "planetary overload" (McMichael 1993) or "overshoot" (Catton 1982). In his review of a wide range of scholarly estimates of the earth's capacity to support population, the demographer Joel E. Cohen concludes:

The human population of the Earth now travels in the zone where a substantial fraction of scholars have estimated upper limits on human population size . . . the possibility must be considered seriously that the number of people on the Earth has reached, or will reach within half a century, the maximum number the Earth can support in modes of life that we and our children and their children will choose to want.

(Cohen 1995a, 342)

Since the human impact on earth represents a combination of resource use, culture, and technology, no definite figure can be given for earth's capacity to support a specific number of people. It is important, however, to take into account the approximate numbers that have been calculated for various levels of consumption. The estimates that Cohen surveyed clustered in the 4–8 billion range (Cohen 1995a, 1995b). Boyden and Dovers noted that perhaps 4–5 billion people could live on earth in a universally agricultural world, while a group at Cornell estimated in the mid-1990s that only 1–2 billion people could live sustainably on earth in "relative prosperity" (Pimentel et al. 1994; Whittaker and Likens 1975). It is unclear whether the world is at or beyond an absolute limit of growth and whether, once the combined curve of population and consumption peaks, the curve will stay at a steady high level, oscillate, or fall steeply. It is clear, however, that since humans have pushed the earth's biosphere close to its carrying capacity, something has to give.

There is an unpleasant arithmetic at work here. On one hand, if global average per-capita consumption falls off while the population curve continues to rise, nature's condition will continue to decline because of increasing population impact, and the number of people living in abject poverty—now estimated to be about a billion—will mushroom. On the other hand, if the population levels off and the average per-capita intensity of resource use continues to increase, the human economy will exhaust the natural world. As the natural world's productive capacity shrinks, living standards and population will decline (Meadows, Meadows, and Randers 1992).

Moral Aspects of Limits

Hovering near the earth's limits is a culturally constraining and uncomfortable place for humanity to be—with poor public health, limited opportunity, social struggle, and almost unavoidable decline. Those already living in abject poverty know something of what being at earth's capacity is like: It is a world of abysmal public health. Average life spans are short and annual death rates exceed birth rates. There is extensive suffering from social instability, natural and human disasters, inadequate public health infrastructure, the march of epidemic diseases, the appearance of new pathogens, and the resurgence of old ones such as tuberculosis and malaria. Pathogens are strengthened and spread by under-nutrition and polluted water. Much of the day's work is spent in fetching water and wood, coping with fatigue, risking exposure to weather extremes, and pursuing education with virtually no books or paper. The capacity for human achievement is necessarily stunted (Homer-Dixon 2000).

Many in these circumstances choose to migrate or are forced to do so by social disruptions and starvation. The 1990s chaos of Rwanda, Burundi, and Zaïre are examples, but an epidemic of migration is present in every major global region. The United States Committee for Refugees estimated in 2002 that the worldwide international refugee population grew to almost 15 million in 2001, while those displaced within their own countries numbered about 22 million (U.S. Committee for Refugees 2002). People are moving to the increasingly crowded and chaotic urban areas of the world, which are therefore growing far faster than overall population. Six and a half billion people are expected to live in cities by 2050, more than all people alive in the world in 2002 (Brown, Gardner, and Halweil 1998, 43).

The world of fundamental scarcity is a world of conflict over life's most basic resources. These conflicts are aggravated by growing global inequalities, international debt, transfer of wealth from the South to the North, and the sale of weapons by wealthy nations to poor (in most years, the United States is the lead marketer of weapons internationally). Populations concentrated in cities, dependent on resources drawn from ever wider geographical ranges, are vulnerable to disruptions in global economic and civil institutions. More mass deaths during famines, social conflicts, earthquakes, floods, storms, heat waves, and epidemics are to be expected.

At minimal levels of survival, even the best public health efforts become self-defeating, because any growth in population resulting from improved public health must only reduce the per-capita resources available to each person. At these minimal levels, public health and quality of life must again decline, a process that Maurice King and Charles Elliott have termed the "demographic trap" (King and Elliott 1993). As natural materials for human welfare become unavailable, sequestering resources for nature restoration comes at an increasingly high cost to neighboring human populations. Forest restoration, for example, must restrict the availability of wood for cooking. As these problems spread, there are fewer opportunities for escape. Sooner or later, the whole planet funnels into a downward population and consumption spiral.

In such a world, the material basis for human freedom evaporates. Individuals lack the material resources necessary to assert a sense of voluntariness in their decisions. They have little capability to produce or command food, clothing, shelter, medical care, contraception, and other resources minimally necessary for an adequate life (Nussbaum and Sen 1993). The degraded natural world provides little enjoyment; there is little hope of advancement. The capacity of society to protect human rights deteriorates.

Here in the present, near the limits of earth's capacity, the commitment of the First World to an upward curve of material growth can only worsen problems for people around the world and deepen the debt charged to nature and future generations by decimated forests, spent fisheries, exhausted topsoil, and a torn and fragmented web of life. The greater the overshoot, propelled in part by the intensity of First World material consumption, the more these problems are aggravated. The longer the First World pursues the trajectory of growth, the more realistic and dire becomes the possibility of collapse.

Sustainability

Major cultural and economic changes are necessary in the First World in order to mitigate these dismal scenarios. The First World needs to switch to a sustainable trajectory—a society shaped by population reduction, significantly reduced consumption, and a commitment to reverse the downward trend in the condition of nature.

The term *sustainability* worked its way into the public vocabulary in 1980, with the publication of Lester Brown's *Building a Sustainable Society* and the International Union of Conservation of Nature's *World Conservation Strategy*. The concept gained widespread recognition from the so-called Brundtland Report, the report of the United Nations Commission on Environment and Development, published in 1987. The Brundtland report emphasized "sustainable development" and reflected a growing international effort to understand global economic development in ecological terms. It was already clear by then that earth's natural systems were under strain. The need for development in the Southern Hemisphere —to overcome widespread poverty—was obvious, but how to achieve it without causing a total collapse of planetary systems poses still-unsolved challenges.

The lack of specificity in the population and consumption growth debate is a conceptual and moral vulnerability in the argument for significant social change: How can we propose policies that respect limits without a clear sense of how to define sustainable limits? If establishing limits now means sacrificing some goods, some material standard of living, is it ethical to act on such a vague articulation of the problem? The paradox of sustainability is that it must remain fluid enough to be philosophically useful and integrative while specific enough to monitor progress.

Although *sustainability* has perhaps suffered from excessive vagueness, much work is being invested in the development of new standards by which to judge the performance of entities with respect to sustainability. New forms of measurement include "life-cycle" and "cradle-to-cradle" analyses of products, a wide variety of measurements of material and energy flow, tracking of the individual household ecological footprint, and gauges of the condition of atmosphere, soil, water, and forest. New forms of economic measurement are being developed to reflect human welfare more accurately than dollar flow (Henderson 1996). Institutions are identifying examples of, and awarding public prizes for, best practices in architecture, design, planning, materials, and product development. Quantified measurements and models like these need wider implementation and public familiarity so that the world can better estimate the limits of natural systems, monitor human pressures on them, and judge the quality of environment and life achieved. Such measures support the hope of evolving toward an optimal balance between the quality of life and stable, sustainable ecosystems.

Creating measurements and identifying models requires communities to define more explicitly what they want to sustain. They must define system boundaries both geographically (should bioregions, cities, nations, or ecosystems be the basis of divisions?) and temporally (do we look for the signs of progress over years, decades, or centuries?). They also must define seemingly objective concepts such as "resources," "scarcity," "growth," and "limits," since these cannot be conceptualized in purely physical terms. Moreover, since the elements of the quality of life are widely contested, the enterprise of setting up reliable measures requires reflection on values and ethics. Although there is controversy over which values are most worth sustaining, the value elements of sustainability cannot be completely arbitrary. They must respect Herschel Elliott's dictum that "an acceptable system of ethics is contingent on its ability to preserve the ecosystems which sustain it" (Elliott 1997).

Elliott's principle makes sustainability itself one of the fundamental elements of ethics. Sustainability assumes that value extends beyond the present, that rich and healthy ecosystems have value both in themselves and as the conditions of human thriving, and that humans, through voluntary choices and programs of action, can change unsustainable practices. The value elements of sustainability are also key, because any new programs necessary to bend the population and consumption curves downward will need to be meaningful to most of the population; otherwise, such efforts are bound to collapse in a relatively short time. Work on ethics is an important part of building cultural change.

Sustainability, Population Limitation, and Public Health

When we discuss the problem of earth's limits with medical students, we hear a recurring refrain:

The problem of population is already solving itself. The spread of HIV, especially in Africa, is shortening life expectancy and reducing fertility. This means that inevitably the human population will come to terms with earth's limits. There is nothing we need to do here in Nebraska about this; we should just continue business as usual.

It is troubling that medical students could fail to notice the cruelty and indifference of this point of view. The spread of HIV in the world, though it does indeed shorten the average human life span, is not the solution to the population problem; it is part of the terror, grief, and human cost of the world's current population-consumption overload. HIV is not part of the solution to growth; it is part of the problem of growth. Such opinions fail to appreciate that the world as a whole is reaching its limits and that these limits cannot be repaired by destroying people and their habitats.

Indifference to poor public health fails to respect obligations that are well understood, particularly in the medical professions, to avoid harm to human well-being now and into the future. Without public health, people lack the personal capabilities to cope with or to turn around the decline in our surroundings. As environmentally generated ills increase, and we react by increasingly turning our resources to materially expensive rescue measures and not prevention, we are likely to erode the environment more swiftly. Although some pro-nature, anti-human enthusiasts may be hoping for diseases and poisons to target humans and spare animals and plants, the decline of human numbers through poor public health surely creates conditions unhealthy for ecosystems as well. Good public health is necessary in order to respect our moral responsibility toward the natural world as well as to ourselves.

Public health needs to be considered not just in terms of its current status, but in the context of our ability to maintain health in the long run. The maximum average "natural" human lifespan is roughly eighty-five years (Olshansky, Carnes, and Cassel 1990), so health planning for just one lifespan covers most of a century, and the best planning includes several generations. This means that normal economic discounting methods cannot be used for public health planning. Repeated discounting by decade reduces the value of future health needs to nearly nothing, when in fact public health needs are relatively stable over centuries at least. Protecting public health is more like building capital than like expending resources (Anand and Sen 1996).

Yet one of the problematic outcomes of good public health is that it increases average lifespan, thereby increasing the need to reduce birthrates to lower levels in order to limit population size. For this reason, we are generally opposed to medical research conducted with the deliberate intention to increase the lifespan, as success in this area would make zero population growth impossible without an absolutely minimal birthrate (Sinsheimer 1978).

In contrast, ethical birth limitation is possible. Many nations are achieving very low growth levels without coercion; indeed, families often seek birth control despite social efforts to discourage them. Improvements in family planning are associated with morally sound social programs such as adequate primary health care, maternal health services, and comprehensive reproductive health services for women. Birth limitation can also be fostered by improving the status of women—creating access to education and employment and encouraging women's rights to negotiate with men on intimate decisions affecting reproduction (Ashford et al. 2002).

People in industrially developed countries tend to think that programs for birth limitation should be fostered primarily in regions where birth rates are higher and where local environmental damage by growing populations is important. But the more a person consumes, the greater the environmental impact of that person's life, so the world's consumers also need to limit births. Low birth rates are every regional culture's obligation, except perhaps for small populations of threatened tribal and language groups who are well integrated with their local ecosystems.

Sustainability and Consumption

Since population size can decline only slowly, the first place we should look to establish sustainability is in limiting consumption—a particular obligation to those who use the most "stuff," the billion or so people of the "consumer class" of the earth. If, as some claim, it is the chief responsibility of the world's poor to have fewer children, it is the chief responsibility of the world's rich to use less of the earth's resources. Consumption is widely viewed in the United States as an innocent pleasure, a social obligation on behalf of the economy, a mark of blessedness, a means of displaying status, and an appropriate reward for success. So it is a puzzle for people to consider that this ordinary satisfaction is actually deeply problematic.

Yet, long before the present environmental crisis, people reflected on the effects of material goods and consumption on individuals, the human spirit, and the social fabric. Historically, consumption has received a mixed review: damning of the wealthy, sermons on frugality, and simple envy can be found throughout history. Many thoughtful spiritual accounts of what is good and meaningful in life share a warning against the excessive love or pursuit of material goods (Durning 1992, 144).

An appreciation of the problematic impact of consumption on the environment has been slow in coming, even though many early civilizations were destroyed when local overexploitation eliminated key resources such as forest and arable land (Ponting 1991). A dominant Western view has been that the work of clearing land, planting fields, and draining swamps is an expression of the human duty to perfect God's creation. This optimistic view did not begin to weaken until the eighteenth and nineteenth centuries, when industrial pollution in Europe and the decimation of North America's pristine wilderness by the European invaders made problems increasingly obvious (Glacken 1967; Marsh 1854). Meanwhile, the celebration of consumption and an appreciation of its value to economic growth spread, abetted by the growth of modern rational philosophies that displaced older conceptions of the meaning of life, celebrating a sense of place, natural cycles, and the abundance of nature as sources of meaning (White 1967).

What is Consumption?

Consumption consists of human and human-induced transformations of materials and energy. Consumption is environmentally important to the extent that it makes materials or energy less available for future use, moves a biophysical system toward a different state or, through its effects on those systems, threatens human health, welfare, or other things people value.

(Stern et al. 1997, 20)

In thinking about how to reduce the environmental impact of consumption, it is useful for our purposes here to distinguish three different levels:

- *Primary consumption* generates most of the impact on the natural world. It includes the processes of extraction, transformation, manufacture, and disposal by which the materials of society are drawn from and returned, greatly changed, to nature. This is the more problematic side of consumption Stern speaks of.
- *Secondary consumption* consists of the items and capital in daily use in the consumer world—cars, computers, tools, beds, pipes, tubes, and so on. This is the end-user side, the "good" side of consumption, the experience of useful or pleasurable items. As with primary consumption, end use also has an immediate impact on nature. For example, building a new suburban hospital may displace woodland, and driving a car emits carbon into the atmosphere.
- *Tertiary consumption* is more abstract. This is the broader concept or value that the material good serves. For example, eating food (secondary consumption) serves nutrition and conviviality; driving a car serves transportation, and building a hospital serves therapy. This is a useful concept of consumption because it allows us to consider that radically different material options might serve similar valued ends. For example, if transportation is at issue, urban regions can replace cars with public transit systems and bicycles. Hospitals can be displaced in part by better public health measures.

Most of the environmental impact of consumption in the First World is incurred at the primary level. By some estimates at least half of the waste and energy cost for most items occurs during manufacture and disposal. The end-user phase of products is only a narrow slice of their full life cycle (Durning 1992, 164 note 8). For technologically complex items such as computers and X-ray machines, the ratios of materials and energy used in primary production to the mass of the end-user object is much higher.

It is neither technologically nor conceptually difficult to imagine a number of ways primary consumption can be reduced without having much impact on secondary consumption. Especially in North America, factories can employ energy more efficiently; homes can be better insulated; cars can be downscaled and made more fuel-efficient; products can be engineered with lighter materials; and products and materials can be reused, reprocessed, and recycled. Similarly, consumers can include environmental criteria in their purchases and demand products with superior environmental features in their manufacture. Millions of people are developing creative ways to implement these changes at all levels of production and consumption.

Yet crucial questions remain: how much reduction in primary consumption is really called for? For example, is the 7% reduction in U.S. atmospheric carbon output proposed by the initial Kyoto protocol enough to do the job? Can all of the work of minimizing the impact on nature be done at the level of primary consumption so that consumers can remain comfortable with their habits, or are significant changes in secondary consumption necessary as well? Can consumption be reduced enough to begin to heal the natural world while people can still continue to meet their basic needs?

Scaling primary consumption. By what scale or factor does the human impact on the earth need to be reduced? In pursuing this question we move squarely into a realm of approximations and guesses based on complex assumptions, such as projections about where global population might level off, a sense of the rate of the decline in the natural world, and estimates of how many species and how much forest and wilderness need to be preserved in order to avoid collapse or a spiritually empty earth. Estimates also depend on whether primary attention is directed to consumer societies or average levels of consumption around the globe as a whole. (The latter neglects the obvious need to treat differently radically different types and levels of consumption in different regions of the world.) Estimates also depend on a sense of how fast changes can be made, since in this rapidly deteriorating situation the longer it takes to turn trends around, the sharper is the turn required to save what remains.

Meadows and her group calculated a decade ago that world throughput would have to level off in the early part of the twenty-first century at about one quarter to one eighth of 1990 levels to avoid a collapse in population and standard of living (Meadows, Meadows, and Randers 1992, and personal communication). (*Throughput* is a general term used to refer to the amount of energy involved in the full life cycle of products from extraction to final disposal of materials.) In 1995, Kauppi estimated that in order to stabilize global climate change, human carbon atmospheric output would probably have to be reduced to one third or less of its then-current levels (Kauppi 1995). In 1994, von Weizsäcker, Lovins, and Lovins introduced the concept "Factor Four"—a hypothetical fourfold increase in resource productivity. They identified fifty technologies, many related to energy, where readily available improvements could quadruple resource productivity. They estimated that overall global throughput would need to be halved during the next fifty years in order to achieve sustainability (von Weizsäcker, Lovins, and Lovins 1995).

Developed around 1990 and since refined by Wackernagel and colleagues, ecological "footprint" analysis (see note 1) is another way to approach this question. Ecological footprint analysis indicates how much land area is required to regenerate biologically what each person uses at a given level of secondary consumption. Wackernagel and his colleagues estimate that, about twenty years ago, throughput began to surpass earth's regenerative capacities, and that current levels of primary consumption exceed supply by about one fifth (Wackernagel et al. 2002). This is a more optimistic estimate, apparently only requiring about a 20% global reduction in average throughput to halt decline.

It is when attention turns to the world's consumer class that the case for reducing consumption becomes most compelling. A substantial proportion of global consumption and consequent harm to the natural world originates from the consumerist economies of the world's developed nations. Estimates of the relative share of the world's resources going to the world's wealthiest vary. The United Nations Population Fund estimates that the richest fifth of the world's people account for over 80% of all private consumption (based on dollars spent), while the poorest fifth of the world's population consumes about 1.3%, for a ratio of about fifty to one (United Nations Population Fund 2001). Durning surveys a range of materials and finds that the quarter of the world's people who live in the most-developed industrialized nations consume anywhere from 40% to 86% of the world's materials. The higher percentages apply to industrial and technical materials, such as steel, chemicals, aluminum, and paper. Energy materials fall into the mid-range at about 60% to 75%, along with timber, meat, and fertilizers. The lower ranges refer to less-processed commodities more closely related to meeting basic needs, such as water, fish, grain, and cement (Durning 1992, 50).

According to the World Wildlife Fund's ecological footprint analysis, the global ecological footprint in 1999 covered 13.7 billion hectares, or an average of 2.3 hectares per person (World Wildlife Fund 2002, 4) (1 hectare = 2.47 acres). While the average Asian or African has a footprint of about 1.4 hectares, the average North American's is about 9.6 hectares, well above the earth's biological capacity of 1.90 hectares per person (Executive Summary). The energy footprint—the fastest-growing component of the global footprint—is also the most unequally divided, with a 16-fold disparity in energy consumption between rich and poor countries (World Wildlife Fund 2002, 14). If everyone in the world were to consume materials and energy at American rates, more than five Earths would be required unless there were radical changes in methods of production (Wackernagel et al. 2002).

Some analysts are optimistic that large-scale changes in the environmental impact of production can be achieved. For example, the Factor Ten Club, an international group working out of the Wuppertal Institute in Germany, calls on industrialized nations to achieve a tenfold increase in energy and resource productivity—a goal they consider well within reach over the next thirty to fifty years (Factor Ten Club 1994). Many businesses that have "greened" their industrial processes have found that they can make large reductions in environmental impact, often at little or no additional cost to their enterprise (Hawken, Lovins, and Lovins 1999; McDonough and Braungart 2002).

Scaling secondary consumption.   Must these needed technological changes affect people's life styles? Can't the engineers take care of the problems? Given the levels of reduction in consumption required, especially in the First World, a good sense of realism would answer that Americans must also make significant reductions in secondary consumption in order to achieve sustainability.

There are limits to efficiency past which machinery just cannot go, especially in areas of energy transformation, which have been thoroughly studied (Peet 1992; Smil 1994). First, molecule for molecule, industrial society continues to be sustained by hydrocarbon because of its heavy use of such materials as wood, paper, plastic, composites, and fossil fuels (Wernick 1996). Efficiency in the use of hydrocarbon materials is already well advanced, so radical reductions are unlikely. Second, the main hope of environmentalists for new energy sources lie in solar and wind power, but to construct a society around these forms of production would greatly change the geography, economics, and interconnections of existing communities. Third, present modes of production are so large in scale and so well entrenched that it would take a great deal more than a new idea to make change. Technological magic will need to be replicated all over the world, and would need to be accompanied by a huge investment in capital, education, and organization. Finally, industrial agriculture already makes heavy demands on limited territory, water, and soil: all proposals to rest production on renewable and natural materials must compete with the already inelastic demands on the land from agriculture. At the same time, genetic modifications to crops can only advance food production within the terms set by the air, soil, and moisture around them (Smil 1991; Brown 1995).

While engineers and economists can reorganize primary consumption, consumers in a financial position to be flexible in their purchases can help. They can send a message to the market by examining the environmental impact of potential purchases and reducing consumption. They can target areas where improvements are easy to achieve: replacing some of the meat in their diets with grain, avoiding toxic products, buying from small, local manufacturers, using more-durable materials, and repairing rather than replacing broken or worn-out goods. Consumers can also reduce the environmental impact of health care by leading healthier lives and using fewer medical products.

Meeting needs.   The current global predicament of poverty is both tragic and unjust. A billion or so people live with much less than they need; many more have just enough, even though there probably is enough food, energy, and materials around the world to meet basic needs were it better distributed. Nevertheless, some may feel that our argument for limiting consumption is too harsh on the First World. More can be extracted from the environment to meet the needs of the world's poor, and it would be unhealthy and harmful for people of the First World to use fewer resources when they are using many of these resources to meet basic needs.

Much of the consumption of the First World is discretionary and not used to meet basic needs. Shrader-Frechette argues that the duty to protect the environment overrides "weak human rights" to low-priority uses of environmental resources. So, First World consumers have a strong obligation to bring the scale of their unneeded secondary consumption way down, or at the very least, to radically reduce the primary consumptive aspects of unneeded consumption (1991). In contrast, Shrader-Frechette also holds that "strong human rights" related to basic survival should take priority over wilderness restoration and species preservation, unless there is danger of ecosystem collapse.

A closer look at how the First World meets its needs suggests that the environmental costs of meeting needs can and should be reduced. Housing is a basic need; yet American houses and apartments are growing in per-capita square footage at significant environmental cost, even though a small apartment or house meets the need for shelter. Transportation is a basic need, but sport utility vehicles are, for most of those who drive them, unnecessarily large and inefficient. As David Brooks points out, many well-off Americans have fallen into the trap of "extravagant utility," where they feel obligated to meet their needs with the highest-status products (Brooks 2000).

Good health, of course, depends directly on consumption (food, water, adequate shelter, etc.), but the tempting conclusion that more consumption equals more health does not follow. The consumption of too much food, for example, leads to obesity, diabetes, heart disease, and stroke; consumption of fatty foods may also contribute to cancer risks. In the last two decades, the United States has experienced an epidemic of obesity and a consequent increase in health problems (Flegal et al. 2002; Ogden et al. 2002). Observers note that U.S. consumers waste about one-fourth of the food they buy. Other examples of overconsumption adverse to health abound, many of them obvious, such as alcohol, tobacco, guns, pharmaceuticals, and so on.

McMichael, Woodward, and van Leeuwen offer an illuminating account of the complex relationships between energy use and population health. Increasing energy consumption has been a marker of an improving material standard of living—correlating roughly with a population's life expectancy. At some point, however, the curve of life expectancy as correlated with energy use levels off and then declines. The authors make a convincing case that the industrialized nations have passed the peak; continued growth in consumption is doing more harm than good to health. The most direct effects come from air pollution in urban areas contributing to respiratory infections, bronchitis, asthma, and lung cancer (see also Pope et al. 2002). Indirect effects may be felt from climate change, with its attendant health implications, and acid rain. Energy overconsumption in the industrialized world also has a significant negative impact on the health of populations in the developing world: for example, most of greenhouse gas emissions come from the Northern Hemisphere; yet climate change is likely to be felt most keenly by vulnerable populations in the South (McMichael, Woodward, and van Leeuwen 1994). So, both health and justice can be served by reducing First World levels both of unneeded consumption and meeting basic needs. We will apply this point in the next chapter when we discuss the environmental costs of providing health care.

Conclusion

Any global efforts to address the population-consumption problem must involve:

- Adequate global public health combined with family planning and reproductive health;
- Modest levels of consumption globally;
- New productive technologies and efficiencies;
- An emphasis on meeting needs at low environmental cost; and
- Increased economic equality.

Although it is clear that there must be limits to the growth of population, to consumption, and to damage to the earth's biosphere, societies can and must continue to grow in their ability to satisfy key human values, such as community, equality, health, safety, and education. Since all of these can thrive despite, and perhaps because of, reductions in the scale of consumption, incompatibilities between respect for earth's limits and human welfare are not inevitable.

Many assume that the global economy requires material growth in order to thrive. But the point of an economy is not simply to grow larger; the point is to serve human and natural welfare in the long run. And adjusting economies to support simpler lives provides at least as many opportunities to lead moral lives as do materially more complex lives.

There is an epistemological bottom line central to this argument: Even if there is some doubt that environmentalists' worrisome predictions are correct, it is much more probable that the environment is in danger than that a high level of consumption is necessary for human happiness. Indeed, the latter claim is empirically false as is shown by the literature on happiness (Argyle 1987). There is little of moral worth or essential value that is maintained by a high level of consumption (Singer 1996), while the dangers of excessive consumption are considerable.

Does it follow that U.S. health care needs also to think of a materials revolution and reduction in scale? This question provides our next topic for reflection.

Note for Chapter 3

1. Combined Effects of Population and Consumption

There are several ways to indicate the scale of the human impact on the environment as a result of the combination of population and consumption. One cannot look solely at how population size affects the environment, nor can one consider consumption alone. One needs to look at the numbers (population), how much each individual uses (consumption), how societies as a whole extract and dispose of resources, and the number of people consuming certain amounts. There are four common ways to indicate impact: (a) IPAT, (b) carrying capacity, (c) ecological footprint, and (d) environmental space.

(a) $I = P \times A \times T$

$I = P \times A \times T$ is a formula used to determine human impact on the environment where I is the environmental impact, P is the population size, A is affluence or the level of consumption, and T is level of technological development. Although one could plug numbers into this formula, its key purpose is to underline the dependency of the environmental impact on these particular material features of society. The equation has been challenged for failing to consider less-material aspects of society, such as its economic arrangements, educational levels, or class structure.

(b) *Carrying capacity*

The point at which a population's growth is limited by its environment—by lack of food and space—is called by demographers the "carrying capacity" of the environment. If a population exceeds carrying capacity, it may soon follow a downward curve, where instead of easing off gradually into slow growth, the population crashes, either becoming extinct or maintaining small numbers until conditions are again suitable for growth. Because the concept was used to describe animal populations before it was applied to humans, the term is offensive to some people. In any case, carrying capacity is not the best way to characterize impact because it does not account for consumption levels or quality of life. It refers solely to the number of humans inhabiting a given ecosystem.

(c) *Ecological footprint*

The idea of an ecological footprint conceptualizes the quantity of resources an average person in a defined population uses in terms of the land area needed to produce those resources and recycle the waste from them (Wackernagel and Rees 1996, 9). Although there are difficulties involved in making the concept precise, Wackernagel and Rees have developed a reasonable scheme for calculating footprints (you can estimate your own ecological footprint online at *www.rprogress.org*). The footprint scheme is concerned with the active biological capacity of earth's biomes to accommodate growing crops, grazing animals, harvesting timber, fishing, and burning fossil fuels (expressed as the ability of the earth to sequester carbon released into the atmosphere). This concept helps emphasize the consumption side of overpopulation: populations who consume less can afford larger numbers without exceeding earth's capacity. The most recent outline of the concept can be found in Wackernagel et al. (2002), which also surveys some alternate measures of global human impact.

(d) Environmental space

Environmental space—or "environmental utilization space" in a more literal translation from the Dutch—is usually credited to J.B. Opschoor. It builds on the idea that the biosphere has a limited capacity to provide its services (sources and sinks) at any given point in time. Environmental space underlines the need to set quantified targets for sustainable use of resources and create performance indicators to measure whether we are moving in the right direction. For each indicator (e.g., consumption of land, materials, energy, water, and marine resources) we need to know the current status and have a benchmark value for each. As described by Chambers, Simmons, and Wackernagel, "it is essentially a 'distance to target' approach where sustainable use for key environmental resources is defined as a global target for sustainability" (2000, 21). Environmental space emphasizes inputs (resource consumption) and strongly emphasizes global equity, since a recognition of global limits forces us to face how environmental space is allocated between nations and regions (Hille 1997).

4

Environmental Aspects of Health Care

A collection of fine early nineteenth-century prints by the German artist Karl Bodemer hangs along the brightly lit hallways of the Nebraska Health System's eight-story north campus hospital. These images of Native Americans, elk, and Nebraska's prairies not far in space or time from where the hospital now stands are an evocative contrast to the white coats, industrial glass and tile, and sharp fluorescent lights of the surrounding hospital. The people and animals depicted in the prints are mostly gone now, and the transformation of the Great Plains invites us to ask how long the seemingly sturdy structures of the medical center will continue to thrive. Our brief reflection in this chapter suggests that in its current form health-care is environmentally damaging and that its long-term viability is therefore uncertain.

The health-care system significantly damages the environment—by the overall material scale of its activities and by the variety, toxicity, and volume of its waste stream. Although hospitals represent only one part of the health care system, they are our focus in this chapter because they are so visible and symbolic of healthcare, and because they provide opportunities for organized solutions to environmental problems.

Hospitals operate under complex regulations that address many environmental aspects of medical products and facilities, but clinicians, patients, and ethicists have only recently begun to actively include environmental concerns in their decisions about clinical materials and practices. We are a long way from addressing, in any substantial way, the grave environmental concerns discussed in the two previous chapters. An adequate response to these problems will necessarily involve reductions in the toxicity and volume of health-care materials.

If reducing the environmental impact of health care is to avoid a radical decline in the quality of services, new techniques will have to be found to increase medicine's environmental efficiency. It is unlikely that gains can be made unless medical and basic science research programs deliberately explore ways to reduce the environmental costs of saving lives and reducing suffering. Although some argue that clinicians dedicated to patient care should disregard matters of cost, environmental (not to mention economic) limits must circumscribe the scope of what can responsibly be undertaken in health care, as in the larger economy. Fortunately, professional codes of ethics are beginning to reflect this increased sense of responsibility for the environmental as well as financial costs of health care.

Environmental Problems of Health Care

In 1993, George Simbruner published a one-page statement entitled "Ecological Impact of Pediatric Intensive Care." Simbruner summarized data on his investigation of waste production and resource consumption from his own pediatric intensive care unit (PICU). He estimated the waste caused by the use and disposal of several medical products and their packing materials. A typical Viennese ten-bed PICU, he estimated, would generate waste consisting of about 4000 syringes and a similar number of gloves per week, and 10,000 large waste bags containing medical products, packaging materials, glass, and hazardous waste per year. He noted that these wastes reflect only a small portion of the total amount and variety of materials and toxic chemicals used in making these products (Simbruner 1993). In a similar dive into the trash, two Michigan surgeons estimated waste from five common types of surgical procedures and found weights per procedure ranging from 8.5 pounds for a hernia repair to 43.01 pounds for a heart revascularization (Tieszen and Gruenberg 1992).

Simbruner recommended that environmental damage from medical waste should be a concern for those who care for the health of children: "Pediatric activists, caring for children, do have a responsibility to avoid all ecological damage to the world, which these children are going to inherit" (Simbruner, 1993).

As these analyses suggest, the delivery of health care in an industrialized society has complex and far-reaching ecological reverberations. Industrialized health care in the developed nations requires large quantities of fossil fuels, plastics, medicinal plants, electricity, water, chemicals, minerals, paper, and concrete. The production, distribution, use, and disposal of health-care-related materials composes a portion of the overall ecological burden of all nations, especially of those in the First World. Although the environmental and social costs of the vast and complex network of material and energy flow of health-care materials has not been studied in detail, it is possible to offer general indications of how the environmental problems of health care are like and unlike those of other industries.

Health care employs about one in nine workers in the United States and represents over 13% of the gross domestic product (GDP). Delivering patient care are about 7000 hospitals, 10,000 home care companies, 20,000 long-term care facilities, and over 300,000 medical and dental offices and clinics. Other facilities include chiropractic and osteopathic offices, imaging services, dialysis clinics, family planning clinics, laboratories, and other specialized activities (Davies and Lowe 1999).

Open and functioning all the time, and needing to provide stable, protective environments for patients, U.S. hospitals contrast with most other large buildings in the intensity of their energy consumption for heating, cooling, and air filtering. Because of diverse power, water, and information needs, the construction of hospitals is complex (the next time you pass by hospital renovations or get down into the basement, note the ceiling spaces crowded with pipes and conduits). Medical centers are usually surrounded by parking lots and service buildings that interfere with water flow, stifle vegetation, and reflect heat. The esthetics of academic medical centers seldom include substantial green spaces.

Hospitals generate uniquely complex and hazardous solid, air, and water emissions, including toxic, infectious, allergenic, and radioactive wastes. They use massive technical devices, such as X-ray and magnetic resonance imaging machines, with elaborate production histories, geographically diverse environmental sources, high-energy inputs, and special building infrastructure requirements, such as heavy bracing and lead-lined walls. Hospitals increasingly use robots, scanners, computers, and other information technology with similarly complex environmental histories and futures. Because medical technology generally advances at a rapid pace, there is a correspondingly rapid and costly obsolescence of capital equipment.

Let us consider some of these environmental problems in more detail by grouping them under the two headings "downstream" and "upstream." Downstream effects tend to be the more obvious: what happens to materials and tools after clinicians and patients toss them into wastebaskets or recycling bins, place them in needle or hazardous waste containers, or pour them down the drain. Upstream concerns are those involving extracting and processing materials, and their manufacture, packaging, and distribution before they reach the hospital.

Downstream Effects

The environmentally problematic outputs of hospitals gained public attention as long ago as the 1960s, when medical needles, syringes, and empty prescription bottles began washing up on eastern U.S. beaches and when a number of other medical waste accidents were widely reported in the media. Since then, public concern, coupled with increasing regulatory and economic constraints, has pushed health-care institutions to review their waste streams. Still, no one knows exactly how much medical waste the United States produces each year since few hospitals track this carefully and aggregates are not regularly reported. Estimates range between 2.1 and 4.8 million tons per year, or between 16 and 23 pounds per bed per day (Rutala, Odette, and Samsa 1989). These figures are based on an estimated number of hospital beds and so do not include sources of waste such as clinics, nursing homes, and home-based care.

The waste stream includes office paper, food waste, IV bags, gauze bandages, syringes, human tissues and organs, pharmaceuticals, cytotoxic agents used in chemotherapy, heavy metals such as mercury, and radioactive wastes. General hospital waste usually becomes part of the municipal waste stream and is either sent to a landfill or incinerated. Hazardous and radioactive wastes, which are highly regulated, will typically be transported to a long-term storage facility where they remain either indefinitely or until they are shipped elsewhere, perhaps abroad.

Infectious or "red bag" waste, which makes up about 10% to 15% of the total, is typically incinerated (burned at high temperatures) or autoclaved (treated with very hot steam). Of the two options, autoclaving appears to be environmentally preferable, although the sheer volume of waste is not reduced as it is during incineration. Incomplete sterilization can occur if procedures are followed incorrectly, and some landfill operators have been reluctant to accept the sterilized red bag waste out of fear that pathogens may remain active.

Long the preferred method of disposal, incineration is environmentally problematic largely because inhaling toxic chemicals is one of the more dangerous forms of environmental exposure. Incinerator emissions contain a variety of toxic pollutants, such as cadmium, arsenic, nickel, lead, chromium, dioxins, furans, and several volatile organic compounds. The high percentage of plastics in the hospital waste stream—at least 20% of the total, and about three times the proportion of plastic found in municipal waste—makes incineration particularly problematic. Many plastics in clinical use have a high chlorine content, and a strong body of evidence links burning chlorinated hydrocarbons with high levels of dioxin emissions. Polyvinyl chloride (PVC), the plastic used in intravenous bags and tubing, is a particular object of concern because of its high chlorine content and its significant use in health care. Even though hospitals burn a smaller volume of waste than municipal incinerators and so account for less overall toxic pollution, emission levels of toxic compounds from hospital incinerators tend to be proportionately higher. Dioxins (a family of several hundred compounds of which *dioxin*, or 2,3,7,8-tetrachlorodibenzo-*p*-dioxin (TCDD), is one of the most problematic) are thought to pose the most significant cancer risk associated with incinerator emissions (see note 1). Because hospital incinerators are often located nearby patients and the public, local effects are of key importance.

For at least two decades, environment and health activists and professional organizations have been concerned about the serious and unresolved environmental and human health problems associated with hospital waste. The largest, and currently most active, leader in this area is Health Care Without Harm (HCWH), a network of over two hundred organizations including the American Hospital Association, the American Nurses Association, and the American Medical Association. HCWH has advocated the elimination of mercury from health-care products (see note 2). The organization has sought to keep PVC plastics out of red bag waste, since incinerating PVC creates dioxins. In 1996, responding to HCWH's concerns, the American Public Health Association called for a phase-out of PVC in medical devices because of its link to the creation of dioxins. HCWH has also, more recently, expressed concern about patient exposure to a chemical called di-ethylhexyl-phthalate (DEHP). DEHP is used as a softening agent in otherwise hard PVC, but it tends to leach out from bags and tubes into IV solutions. DEHP is carcinogenic, according to recent studies cited by HCWH. Young children and patients receiving long-term or intense IV procedures appear to be most at risk (HCWH 2002).

Pharmaceuticals and biological products also pose environmental hazards. Some pharmaceuticals and their bodily metabolites are appearing more frequently in U.S. water sources, in which tests find traces of caffeine, codeine, acetaminophen, ibuprofen, fluoxetine, cimetidine, and digoxin. Many antibiotics, steroids, and hormones can also be detected in ground water, but the main sources of these are agricultural rather than medical (Kolpin et al. 2002). According to some reports, drugs broken down in the body may become reactivated by sewage treatment processes. Conceivably, drugs could react with each other in the water supply and create unpredictable dangers. Testing to identify and measure the panoply of pharmaceuticals that might occur in water sources is only beginning to be developed. (Glaspey, Johnson, and Jameton 2003)

Upstream Effects

Once one accepts a sense of responsibility for what flows downstream, it takes only a small logical step to see that moral responsibility flows upstream as well. Those active in reducing the downstream impact of consumption quickly realize that the best way to reduce the quantity and hazardousness of waste is to move further back in the production cycle and thereby ensure that products are made so that they can be reused, reprocessed, and disposed of as harmlessly as possible. This is sometimes termed "pollution prevention" or "P2."

Less is known about the upstream impacts of the health-care sector than about downstream impacts. The material constituents of health-care services rest on an extensive foundation of natural resources, such as basic and rare metals, wood, plant fibers, plant-based pharmaceuticals, rubber, petroleum, water, and so on.

Precursors of health-care products intermingle with materials and processes headed into other forms of consumption, such as transportation and agriculture, so the upstream effects of health care are entangled with those of other economic sectors. The extraordinarily diverse array of raw materials that are eventually transformed into the materials for a clinic visit or a surgical procedure come from all over the world. Both the substances themselves and the trade and production involved in producing and trading them appear to have protracted impacts on human and natural communities (see note 3).

Resources for the Future, a Washington-based think tank, has published a broad overview of the research on the upstream environmental effects of the health-care sector (Davies and Lowe 1999). Pierce and Kerby (1998; see also note 3) isolate one common hospital product and provide a broad life-cycle account of the global environmental impacts associated with the estimated 12 billion latex gloves used annually in U.S. hospitals. Ryan, Durning, and Baker (1997) model a potential paradigm for presenting the environmental aspects of hospital products with their vivid analysis of the upstream impacts of such common products as computers, tennis shoes, and hamburgers. More research of these kinds will contribute to a better understanding of health care's upstream impact.

Reducing the Scale of Health Care

Although more might be done to refine the manufacture and disposal of health care products so that these processes become less toxic, the most direct way to reduce the environmental impact of health care is to reduce the scale of its clinical activities, and thereby reduce the overall quantity of general waste and toxic materials that accompany providing health care. Patients, businesses, policymakers, and scholars have already criticized the magnitude of the U.S. health care system. The call for cost reduction is not, so far, a response to the environmental crisis, but to a crisis of rising financial costs that has been unfolding for three decades (Shi and Singh 1998, 447) In contrast to other developed countries, which spend 8% or 9% of their GDP on health care, the United States spends over 13%. Even more striking, over 40% of all of the dollars spent in the world on health care is used by the United States on its 5% to 6% of the world's population (World Bank 1993, 4).

Health care is straining the ability of payers to budget for it. The roughly $1.3 trillion U.S. health-care system costs the average American consumer over four thousand dollars a year (Levit et al. 2002). This is a challenge for workers, but it is also a challenge for employers who increasingly compete in a global market where other workers receive more modest benefits, often through a public program. Cost is a factor in the difficulties the United States has in finding the taxes to make health insurance available to all citizens, especially after the taxpayer revolt of the 1980s and 1990s and the economic recession at the turn of the twenty-first century.

The costs of health care are expected to continue to increase significantly. The demand for services is likely to increase as the "baby boomers" age. Pharmaceutical costs are also likely to rise, as companies invest heavily in a new generation of drugs that use molecular and genetic technologies. These will be expensively created drugs on which the pharmaceutical companies expect to recover their investment.

Many patients and clinicians are poorly served by the large industrial facilities, long waiting times, understaffed services, extensive paperwork, complex insurance programs, and the impersonal atmosphere of large-scale corporate health care. Some also charge that payments for health care are increasingly and unfairly directed toward top-heavy administrative expenses and marketing costs, and that too much is invested in the more highly paid professionals such as physicians, while hospitals are understaffed by poorly paid nurses and aides. Others worry that the large U.S. investment in tertiary health care services undermines investment in public health services (Evans 1994).

As Dan Callahan has pointed out, the unsustainable scale of health care pervades all its activities (1998). Using the financial crises suffered by health-care systems around the world during the 1990s as evidence, Callahan argues that modern medicine, in its present form, is unsustainable. Resting on a misguided notion of infinite progress, it is too large and too expensive. Glamorizing highly specialized and technologically advanced acute-care medicine, it neglects many of the health needs of patients. In reaching for its unrealistic goals it threatens its own viability.

If the U.S. economy needs to be scaled down in order to be sustainable, it follows that the health-care system must be scaled down as well. How much reduction in scale should we expect of health care if technically advanced care moves toward sustainability? From a practical point of view, the health-care sector cannot be neatly isolated; basic sources of energy, buildings, materials, transportation, roads, water, and so on, serve health care and connect it deeply with the rest of the economy. If the economy were significantly redesigned for sustainability, health care would be unable to remain anywhere near its present scale or form. And as we argued in the last chapter, sustainability may require reductions in the material and energy throughput of the U.S. economy on the order of half, three quarters, or more. If the rest of the economy were to shrink, for example, by half, without any corresponding contraction of health care, the health-care system would consume an imprudent 26 percent of the economy. So, if other industrialized nations are spending something closer to the "right" proportion of their economies on health care (8% or 9%), then health care would need to shrink by perhaps three quarters in order to match a halving of the United States overall throughput.

Using Dollars to Assess Proportions

An objection can be made to these rough estimates that financial or "dollar" costs inaccurately reflect environmental costs, which are normally "externalized" from corporate accounting. Percentage of GDP is a poor indicator of environmental scale. Some environmentally friendly practices may be financially expensive; for example, installation of photovoltaic cells to collect solar energy may offer environmental savings but cost more than coal-fired plants rated at an equivalent electrical output. In contrast, many efforts to reduce the costs of health-care supplies have resulted in increased environmental costs, such as switching to disposable linens, gowns, bed liners, and surgical tools.

Health care may be environmentally less costly than its share of the GDP would indicate, but we can only guess at this point, since the environmental costs of health care have not yet been assessed in any coherent fashion and since environmental assessments of other sectors are still young. Health care is labor-intensive, and labor costs, since they support people and not environmentally damaging technologies, do not necessarily cause environmental harm. Health care is also a knowledge industry, and the environmental costs of developing, storing, and distributing knowledge are perhaps relatively low. It is possible, then, that while the U.S. economy contracts materially, the shrinking of health care may not need to be as great as the dollar proportions seem to suggest.

Can Health Care Be Ethically Reduced in Scale?

One might object that shrinking our technologically grand conception of health care is neither practical nor ethical. A materially large system feels safe as a psychological bastion against death, suffering, and disease. It is more comfortable for environmentalists who support simple living to imagine building smaller houses and traveling by public transit, which promise more health benefits than hazards, than to consider limiting throughput in the more sensitive arena of health care. But if the scale of health care in the United States remains intensive over the next decades, health care will inevitably suffer increasing shocks as the cost of resources and waste disposal rises and the number of patients suffering from environmentally related diseases grows. Services will become increasingly irrelevant to health-care needs, and costs will more clearly drain the resources needed to restore a healthy environment.

The mirage of modern medicine (to use René Dubos's image) is one facet of the dream of progress as increasing material comfort and mastery over nature, a dream that is drifting into nightmare. The expansionist mindset strives for the gradual and eventually perfect victory over disease, disability, and perhaps even aging and death. While in this dream state, medicine remains oddly oblivious to the large-scale constraints of ecosystems. "Sustainability is specifically useful in calling attention to the need for a medicine that does not require constant progress or unlimited horizons to be humanly valuable, and which may in fact be harmed by them" (Callahan 1998, 34).

Medical Research

Some of those who address environmental issues believe that research and technology will more or less inevitably find ways to solve the environmental problems of production, so that researchers will not need to make deliberate changes in the direction of medicine. Julian Simon and other cornucopians argue that humans, being infinitely ingenious, will be able to shift to new areas for the exploitation of nature when old ones have been played out (Simon and Kahn 1984). Because medicine raises such deep and passionate hopes, challenging the value or direction of health-care research is more difficult in health care than in other social realms.

But history and archeology tell a different story. Many societies have come to an end after destroying their environmental foundations without finding technical solutions to their problems (Ponting 1991). Even if sustainable medical technological ideas were ready on the shelf, technological salvation is not just a matter of having a good idea. That idea must be built and distributed, and such distribution is by no means inevitable, especially as the technological metabolism of First World industry is, in aggregate, unsustainable. And if, as enthusiasts of unfettered technological development claim, technology will save everyone, why has it not already saved the present billion or so poor from undernourishment, starvation, and absolute poverty?

Not only does the cornucopian position fail to show even the slightest regret for the great losses to nature already incurred, it fails to recognize that production has become dependent on the single natural resource of fossil fuel for energy and materials. In our lifetime we have seen metal, fiber, stone, cloth, leather, bone, and wood replaced by fossil-fuel based functional equivalents. Industrial society is becoming a one-resource society, ever more vulnerable to the instabilities of increasing production costs, climate change, and conflicts over sources of extraction (Klare 2001). Industrial health care is particularly dependent on plastics and chemicals, and so, rather than being secure from the larger problems of industry, its capacity to serve is more likely to suffer from the limits of the earth than other areas of consumption.

Even where pharmaceuticals are drawn from renewable sources such as trees and plants, we may encounter environmental obstacles. Some scientists have argued the need for saving rainforests and other pristine areas in order to protect potential sources for new medical products. But to find a rare plant and to use it in medicine may put plants and habitat at risk of over-exploitation. And if we avoid this outcome by finding an alternative synthesis from fossil fuels, we then return to that source dependency. Researchers are working on plans for forest management to protect diversity with controlled production, but such projects can by no means result from undirected research only; they require deliberate policy decisions.

Two Cultures in Biological Research (Snow 1993)

Bench scientists commonly have a different idea of nature than wildlife biologists do. It is our general impression that those wildlife biologists who spend their time in wild areas where they observe rapid changes resulting from the destructive advance of industrial society, worry about the state of nature. Many are in despair. In contrast, medical researchers and bench scientists seem to us, on the whole, to take a more optimistic view. For the latter, "nature" signifies the "laws of nature," which can never be threatened or extinguished. Since medical scientists have dedicated their lives to laboratory work in the hope that they can cure diseases and reduce suffering, environmental problems are sometimes disregarded as outside their sphere of concern. Despite this cultural barrier, many bench scientists doing medical research—toxicologists and cancer specialists, for example—are vocally concerned about the health and environmental costs of industry.

Complementary and Alternative Medicine

It is indicative of this cultural chasm that the field of bioethics has tended until recently to avoid the subject of complementary and alternative medicine (CAM) and to focus more on the ethical problems of allopathic medicine. The reason is primarily political and not conceptual: ethicists making their way in the medical environment are expected to keep their work relevant to the institutional setting, and, often, not to rock the boat. Discussions of CAM—yet another unpopular topic in clinical circles—is a sure road to egregious career risks for bioethicists.

Yet when we describe our concerns about the environmental costs of health care, CAM is often the first concept that leaps to people's minds as an environmentally preferable alternative to conventional health care. CAM is a primary area in which critics of medicine who are concerned with nature and environmental values have developed their ideas. It provides widespread cultural support and appealing rationales for engaging in less environmentally costly lifestyles, countering consumerism, living healthy lives, and encouraging individual responsibility. Together with groups advocating simple living, CAM can do much to reduce the upstream scale of consumption.

Yet, the readily available literature on CAM appears to overlook the environmental costs of the whole life cycle of CAM health products. The push for organic food products is perhaps where the upstream side of CAM is most highly developed, but not many accounts of herbs, vitamins, or homeopathic concoctions go beyond questions of toxicity to consider the scale of production, the distances products travel, costs of packaging, and the costs of disposal.

What, for example, would be the consequences of switching, where possible, from fossil-fuel based products to cleanly produced CAM equivalents derived from renewable agricultural sources? Consider aspirin, one of the most widespread drugs of the pharmaceutical industry. The United States produces billions of aspirin pills annually from simple fossil-fuel based precursors. The most common renewable source of salicylate used widely before the advent of aspirin was and continues to be willow bark. Disregarding issues of dose and efficacy for a moment, what if we all switched from synthetic aspirin to willow bark? Even if willow bark were harvested on a sustainable basis without killing the trees, how much land area and how many willow trees would it take to displace synthesized aspirin for the treatment of arthritis and mild pain and discomfort? A back-of-the-envelope calculation shows that many millions of acres of new forest area would need to be planted and harvested, in competition with land area already committed to forest and agriculture. And what if plant substitutes were promoted for many other synthetic pharmaceuticals as well? How much forest land would this take? So far, we are unaware of any such estimate. This reflects the depth of the world's current environmental bind: moving from fossil fuels to current living biomass for health care would put increasing pressure on already strained ecosystems—a key reason the doctrine of "use less" makes sense.

High-Tech Medical Engineering

What of the high-tech route? How hopeful should environmentalists be for greener products derived from new molecular and genetic approaches? Some scientists believe that new molecular methods will be helpful because dosages require much smaller quantities of materials. Laboratory testing and medical research has been dematerializing in recent years, but it is important to consider the full life cycle of these new methods. [*Dematerialization* refers to a reduction in the quantity of materials required to create an industrial end product or to serve a particular economic function (Wernick, Herman, and Govind et al. 1996)]. Many of them use large, complex laboratory equipment, requiring long production paths with substantial costs in energy and nonrenewable materials. Achieving the high levels of purity of many of these chemicals requires extensive use of volatile solvents, which may be released into the atmosphere and water supplies.

To the best of our knowledge, no one has yet produced a life-cycle overview of the environmental impact of these new biological forms of pharmaceutical production. New molecular and genetic products may be much like antibiotics and therefore capable of being grown on media that derive from renewable sources, but they will also constitute a next generation of technology that builds on existing materials and products, with all the environmental problems of existing products together with new ones of their own.

Present trends in medical research do not seem to us to be showing much concern for the environmental dangers of high-tech medical products. The work of basic researchers in medical schools is increasingly being shaped by economic forces. Under increasing financial pressure to recover investments in research, pharmaceutical evaluation timelines appear to be shortening. Universities have increasingly undertaken royalty agreements with pharmaceutical companies, with the result that some administrators may be wary of supporting projects that highlight the risks of medications.

New genetically engineered agricultural products have come under widespread criticism by environmentalists for their use well in advance of good studies of their potential consequences; yet related medical products coming down the pike have been spared similar criticism, even though their technological and production paths overlap with agriculture considerably. Like agricultural products, genetically engineered medications will be ingested and capable of unpredictable harm to humans. Some new medications are being "pharmed" agriculturally, with the attendant danger that seeds and crops containing genes that express pharmaceuticals might migrate to nearby farms, animal feed, and food products. And with the rise of a new consumerist eugenics driven by the potential to genetically modifiy children, ethicists should be expressing concern about potential hazards of germ-line therapies to the environment. The current line of research on genetic modification, in the face of the widespread extinction of species combined with genetic products' possible unexpected and uncontrollable hazards, radically violates the precautionary principle.

Some formulations of the principle of nonmaleficence give primacy to avoiding harm over doing good (Beauchamp and Childress 2001). The precautionary principle is one such formulation: it asserts that in certain circumstances it is rational to take steps to prevent possible harm even if all the scientific information is not in. Moreover, the burden of proof must shift so that the safety of a proposed endeavor rather than its potential benefit becomes the main focus of concern.

In the United States, the precautionary principle has been applied for the most part to controversies over scientific innovations such as genetically engineered crops that promise benefits but may cause irreversible harm. It has also been used in debates over regulating potentially toxic pollutants where specific agents have been untested but similar agents in the same chemical family have been shown to be dangerous (Raffensperger, Tickner, and Jackson 1999). Greater caution and more environmental evaluation therefore should be shown in the development of new pharmaceuticals.

Shaping Research Directions

Wherever possible, research should be directed toward addressing the most relevant health problems, and the research itself should be carried out in environmentally sensitive ways. A number of administrative processes are already in place that can be used to help integrate environmental concerns into research. For example, the Institutional Review Boards (IRBs) that oversee human-subject research focus largely on the potential risks to subjects, not risks to the public at large. It is conceivable that they could include environmental risks to subjects in their purview. Similarly, academic scientific review committees and study sections at national funding agencies could increase the weight of environmental criteria in setting priorities on health-care research. Hospital administrations use a variety of committees to assess products for purchasing decisions, and these could increasingly include environmental criteria in their evaluation processes (Jameton, McGuire, et al. 2002).

The National Association of Physicians for the Environment has proposed a number of means to reduce the environmental impact of bench research itself (NAPE 1999). By "greening" research, scientists may find new ways to "green" the innovations of their research as well. The National Institutes of Environmental Health Science have also undertaken policy research on selected aspects of the interrelationship of genetic information and the environment (NIEHS 2003). Additional projects might include:

• Developing pharmaceuticals and supplies that require less energy, toxic solvents and catalysts, and materials to manufacture;
• Creating methods for counteracting high consumption levels;
• Developing measures for estimating the environmental impact of health-care products;
• Conducting research on predictable environmental diseases;
• Conducting policy research on lowering the material costs of health care and public health, and on balancing the quality of care with environmental costs.

Professional Responsibility

Eventually, clinicians will need to make judgements about the environmental consequences of their practices. As HCWH has argued, two important ethical points demand clinicians' respect. First, the basic principle of "do no harm" can be read to imply that if health professionals have a responsibility to avoid harming patients, they have a similar responsibility to avoid harming the health of the public and the environment (www.noharm.org). Second, while casual destructiveness might be an anticipated consequence of less morally worthy enterprises, a higher moral standard is expected of health-care professionals.

Health professionals surely have some responsibility to mitigate the environmental costs of health care. The Canadian Association of Physicians for the Environment makes this responsibility explicit:

While the litany of environmental problems and their implications for health summon physicians to play an active role as educators, researchers, and advocates in preventing disease and protecting human and ecosystem health, CAPE believes that we need to start closer to home, and to live out the principle of *primum non nocere*—first do no harm. The health care sector must ensure that it is not itself contributing to the very environmental problems that need to be addressed.

(CAPE 2003)

Although this explicit attention to the environment is rare among health professionals, a review of the ethics codes and related statements of about 115 health profession organizations suggests that the language and concepts central to environmental responsibility are in many cases already in place. Only a few of the reviewed codes and statements include any explicit reference to a responsibility to protect the environment or to conserve materials. Instead, most of these professional codes express general obligations into which it is easy to read an implied obligation. Such common elements of codes and principles include:

- A general obligation to prevent harm to the public,
- Involvement in community and public efforts on behalf of the general welfare, and
- A general concern for justice or widespread access to public health and health-care services.

For example, the seventh principle of the American Medical Association Principles states:

VII. A physician shall recognize a responsibility to participate in activities contributing to the improvement of the community and the betterment of public health.

(AMA 2001)

Environmentally responsible activities can be construed to be among those "contributing to an improved community," and the concept of *community* may be broadened to include the environment. According to the American Academy of Dermatology,

Physicians' responsibility extends to the community and society, and appropriate publicity regarding physicians' participation in community and civic affairs enhances the stature of the profession.

(AAD 2001)

Dermatologists have a particular environmental concern—ozone depletion—because it relates directly to their realm of treatment.

Public safety is another area of implied environmental responsibilities. For instance, the Academy of Medical-Surgical Nurses states:

The nurse acts to safeguard the patient and the public when health care and safety are affected by the incompetent, unethical, illegal, or inappropriate practice of any person.

(AMSN 2002)

Only about ten of these groups have statements showing explicit concern for the environment or conservation of materials. For example, the 1994 American Association of Respiratory Care Code of Ethics states that respiratory therapists should

Refrain from indiscriminate and unnecessary use of resources, both economic and natural, in their practice.

(AARC 1994)

The International Council of Nurses states:

> The nurse also shares responsibility to sustain and protect the natural environment from depletion, pollution, degradation and destruction.
>
> (ICN 2000)

The American Holistic Nurses' Association code contains a paragraph addressed to the environment:

> The nurse strives to manipulate the client's environment to become one of peace, harmony, and nurturance so that healing may take place. The nurse considers the health of the ecosystem in relation to the need for health, safety, and peace of all persons.
>
> (AHNA 2002)

Probably the most explicit and extensive language is that of the International Association of Biomedical Laboratory Science, which displays a developed experience of some of the technical, regulatory, and scientific aspects of environmental protection. It refers to the employment of International Standards Organization environmental criteria and procedures in laboratories. It also touches on workplace health and safety. And it includes reference to larger issues:

> 4. Protect the environment by conserving natural resources.
> 5. Continuously improve our environmental performance, promote safe transportation of hazardous materials, reduce pollution within our operations, conserve the use of energy, fuel, and water, promote an awareness amongst our global member associations.
>
> (IAMLT 1998)

In addition to basic ethics codes, professions express their societal concerns through statements on specific issues. The American Public Health Association, which still has no official code of ethics, has a variety of statements and an "environment and health" agenda that was made one of the top four policy priorities in 1997 (APHA 2002). In 2001, the World Federation of Public Health Associations general assembly stated its support for international action to eliminate persistent organic pollutants, and two years before, the annual meeting made a statement on the public-health consequences of medical waste. The group has also made statements about global climate change, population, and ecological sustainability (WFPHA 2002).

Despite considerable differences of opinion among physicians about how to weigh environmental concerns at the bedside, the American Medical Association has made policy statements promoting environmental health programs, environmental stewardship, recycling medical materials, and combating global climate change. The American Hospital Association has an agreement with the Environmental Protection Agency (EPA) for a project entitled "Hospitals for a Healthy Environment," with the goals of virtual mercury elimination by 2005 and reduction of waste volume by half by 2010 (Hospitals for a Healthy Environment 2003). Health-professional groups have expressed concerns or launched campaigns on wide variety of specific environmental issues with salient health aspects, such as air pollution (asthma), seat belts (automotive injuries), environmental neurotoxins (autism), nuclear weapons (massive casualties), guns (pediatric injuries), dioxins (multiple health problems), and so on.

Judging from the trend of these statements and the need for environmental concern, every health profession would be well within its professional responsibility to include a statement among its basic ethical principles that expressed some or all of the following concerns:

- Prevent pollution, support clean production, reduce the toxicity of medical materials, and reduce waste volume.
- Conserve materials, energy, and natural capital.
- Protect workplace and neighborhood health and safety.
- Exercise precaution where uncertain health risks exist.
- Restore the global ecological foundations of public health.

Conclusion

In order to progress toward a just and viable world, all societies will need to make major changes in how they provide the materials needed for a good life. As we become more imbued with environmental values and see the world from an ecological perspective, a technologically more modest and less toxic constellation of services will find wider acceptance, and societies will be better able to strike a healthy balance among environmental protection, maintenance of public health, and health-care services. Professional and philosophical ethics will similarly need to accept more responsibility for the environmental implications of, and constraints on, their work. Reshaping values, ethics inquiry, and reconfiguring health services should develop together as mutually enhancing and reinforcing activities.

Notes for Chapter 4

1. Dioxins

As of 1995, medical waste incinerators (MWIs) were the third-largest source of dioxin pollution in the United States, according to the EPA (EPA 2000, 1–14). The term *dioxin* refers to a group of chemical compounds with similar chemical structures and biological characteristics. Hundreds of these compounds exist; they are members of three closely related families: the chlorinated dibenzo-*p*-dioxins (CDDs), chlorinated dibenzofurans (CDFs), and certain polychlorinated biphenyls (PCBs). *Dioxin* is also the common shorthand for a specific compound, 2,3,7,8–tetrachlorodibenzo-*p*-dioxin, or TCDD, the best-studied and most toxic of the dioxins. Dioxin produces effects in animal toxicological studies at levels hundreds and thousands of times lower than do most chemicals; early laboratory tests on TCDD, for example, showed it to be thousands of times deadlier to guinea pigs than arsenic. Dioxins are one of the most potent human toxins. At least trace amounts of dioxin—a few parts per trillion—have been found in the blood of all tested humans.

Dioxins are formed when chlorine comes into contact with heated organic molecules. Major identified sources of dioxins in the United States include combustion, metal smelting and refining, and chemical manufacturing. With the exception of PCBs, dioxins have no commercial use, and PCBs are no longer produced in the United States.

The first major health effect of dioxin was recognized in the 1930s when epidemiologists described a new disorder called *cable haulers' disease*. Male workers chronically exposed to PCBs in electrical cables developed skin lesions. This painful and disfiguring skin disease came to be called *chloracne*, a severe acne-like eruption. The first well-publicized dioxin accident occurred in 1948, when workers at a herbicide plant in Nitro, West Virginia, were exposed to dioxins. Like the cable haulers, exposed workers suffered from moderate to severe chloracne. In 1976, an explosion at a trichlorophenol plant in Seveso, Italy, released a pound of dioxin into the air, causing acute and chronic exposures to high levels of dioxin. The acute exposure killed a number of small animals—dogs, cats, and chickens—and caused an outbreak of chloracne in many children in the region. Epidemiological studies of residents have shown increases in many different cancers. In Taiwan in 1979, about two thousand people ate rice oil contaminated with PCBs and dibenzofurans. Children born to women during the next several years were exposed to large doses of dioxins while in utero. Researchers tracking the children noted signs of developmental delay and abnormal sexual development.

In the 1990s, researchers agreed that dioxin exerts most, perhaps all, of its toxic effects through a protein receptor found in individual cells. Dioxin binds to the receptor, occupying its place; it then binds to DNA in the cell, prompting changes in gene expression. This new model for understanding dioxin's toxicity became the groundwork for a decade-long EPA reassessment of dioxin's health risks. This meant moving away from high-dose studies, investigating instead the effects of dioxin at very low levels of exposure where, perhaps counterintuitively, its toxic potential seems to unfold. Researchers also began to refocus their attention away from cancer and toward dioxin's potential developmental and reproductive toxicity.

Long-term health effects include cancer (Hodgkin's disease, non-Hodgkin's lymphoma, and soft-tissue sarcoma), suppression of the immune system, and increased susceptibility to disease (e.g., adult-onset diabetes). Dioxins are also considered endocrine disruptors: they mimic the action of human hormones, disrupting gland function and organ tissues, such as thyroid, ovaries or testes, and the small intestines, by sending wrong signals or blocking the right ones. Although the teratogenicity (tendency to produce mutations) of dioxin has not been established in humans, mice exposed to dioxin were born with cleft palate and hydronephrosis (a congenital obstruction of the ureter). In infants, dioxin is thought to cause delays in reaching developmental milestones. The effects of dioxin on human reproduction, although imperfectly understood, are thought to be significant.

The EPA estimates that 95% of dioxin intake for a typical person is through food, especially foods containing animal fats—beef and dairy products, as well as fish, eggs, and chicken. Dioxin emissions settle on vegetation and grassland; animals consume the plants; dioxins accumulate in the animal's fatty tissue, which humans then eat. Because dioxin concentrates in fat, it is found in human breast milk.

Dioxin levels in the environment have declined over the past 30 years. Between 1987 and 1995 (the two years during which they collected data), EPA estimates that dioxin emissions decreased by 81 percent. With even tougher regulations in place for municipal waste incineration (since 1995) and medical waste incineration (1997), the EPA anticipates a greater than 95% reduction from these two categories, historically the largest industrial sources of dioxin release (EPA 2000). (Sources: National Center for Environmental Assessment 2000, 2001; Bunch 1999; Colburn, vom Saal, and Soto 1993)

2. Mercury

Mercury has been clinically useful because of its uniform response to changes in temperature and pressure. It can be found in a large number of common health-care products and instruments, such as thermometers, sphygmomanometers, gastrointestinal tubes, feeding tubes, esophageal dilators, dental amalgam, laboratory fixatives, pharmaceutical supplies (e.g., contact lens solution), batteries, lamps (fluorescent, germicidal, and ultraviolet), electrical equipment, thermostats, bleach, and vaccines.

Exposure to mercury is dangerous: it can cause permanent damage to the brain, kidneys, and the developing fetus. Symptoms of damage to the central nervous system may include tremors, impaired vision, memory problems, irritability, changes in vision or hearing, and paralysis. Whether vaporized in the atmosphere or deposited into wastewater, mercury eventually makes its way into lake sediment and waterways, where it is converted by microscopic organisms into its most lethal and toxic form: methyl mercury.

The likeliest routes of exposure for humans are eating methyl-mercury–contaminated fish (over forty states post fishing advisories); inhaling inorganic mercury vapors from spills, incinerators, and industries that burn mercury-containing fuels; ingesting mercury from dental work and medical treatments; and absorbing it through skin contact at work; for example, at health-care laboratories. According to the EPA, the most vulnerable populations are women of childbearing age and young children.

Additional sources of mercury pollution include incinerators, coal combustion, cement kilns, and the manufacture of chlorine. Hospitals are the fourth-largest source of atmospheric mercury pollution, from the incineration of mercury-containing products. They contribute between 4% to 5% of the total mercury wastewater load. (Sources: Harvie 1999; Montague 1998; Agency for Toxic Substances & Disease Registry 1997.)

3. Latex Gloves

Latex is a form of natural rubber extracted from the trunk of *Hevea brasiliensis* and other rubber-bearing trees grown on plantations in Malaysia, Indonesia, and Thailand. Over the years, growers have used a combination of chemical ethylene-based stimulants, pesticides, and herbicides on the bark to stimulate latex flow and increase the yield. Chemicals that fall into this category are 2,4–D, PCBs, DDT, 2–4–5–T, and ethylene oxide. On some plantations, protective clothing is used minimally, if at all. Many plantation workers live without adequate access to safe drinking water, food, shelter, sanitation, or health care.

From the extraction of the raw materials through shipment of the final product, transportation of gloves requires a vast network of ships, airplanes, trains, and trucks. Each glove is packed with 99 others inside a cardboard box, which is placed with nine other small boxes inside a case. Cases are loaded into 40-foot ocean containers. Once gloves arrive in the United States, they travel by diesel-powered trains to distribution centers scattered throughout the United States. After a glove is used (often only for a few minutes), it is thrown away into a red bag waste receptacle where it is incinerated, autoclaved, or microwaved. The ash or sterilized waste material is trucked to a nearby landfill and dumped.

Glove use over the years has increased as a result of "Universal Precautions" of the Centers for Disease Control, recommending that health-care workers protect themselves from HIV, hepatitis-B, and other blood-borne pathogens. Over 12 billion gloves were used in 1994 in American Hospital Association registered hospitals—two gloves for almost every person alive on earth. This figure does not include glove use in non-hospital health facilities.

The last few years have seen a push toward latex-free hospital environments since latex allergies are on the rise, with more than 12% of health-care workers experiencing allergic reactions ranging from mild dermatitis to severe anaphylaxis. Synthetic gloves have emerged as the safer alternative, but they, too, have their own set of environmental and human health impacts (Pierce and Kerby 1998).

5

The Green Health Center

What would it be like to establish environmentally sound and sustainable health-care institutions in the United States? What services would ecologically friendly medicine offer? On what scale? What might its guiding ethical principles be?

By developing a hypothetical mission statement and ethical principles for an environmentally sound health-care institution—a "Green Health Center" (GHC)— we can focus on many of the issues that need to be considered in redesigning health care. We can also begin to test, with a concrete (albeit imaginary) example, how to think of an environmentally sound and ethically responsible health care system.

Introducing the Green Health Center

Many major institutions, from universities, to corporations, to hospitals, formulate a statement of mission or vision and an internal code of ethics to guide both the organization as a whole and its individual members. Over the past thirty years, a number large and small businesses in the United States and elsewhere have taken the need for sustainability seriously and have transformed both how they think and how they do business (Freeman, Pierce, and Dodd 2000). Increasingly, businesses have referred to "the environment" in their mission statements, and although some statements are only window-dressing, other corporations have become models of embodied sustainability, with closed loops of production, nearly zero waste, and almost complete energy self-reliance (McDonough and Braungart 2002; Hawken, Lovins, and Lovins 1999). Hospitals, academic medical centers, small clinics, nursing homes, and all manner of other health-care institutions should be able to find similarly creative ways to transform their practices.

To explore how principles of sustainability might transform health-care institutions, a group of scholars and clinicians at University of Nebraska Medical Center developed a mission statement for a hypothetical "Green Health Center." (See Acknowledgements for a list of GHC Working Group members). The Working Group built its conception from the ground up rather than referring to any existing health-care institution. Although environmental considerations eventually must apply to all forms of productive activity—to the entire range of social organizations supporting health and other community activities, from food supply and public health measures to health-care delivery—the Working Group focused on the idea of a single, free-standing health-care center.

As they envisioned it, the Green Health Center would start out small, as a set of clinics providing primary and specialty care. It might also include a hospital and emergency department. For simplicity, the group did not consider nursing homes, long-term care, or psychiatric services, although these also pose important issues and advantages related to our concerns here. The GHC would be managed on a cooperative or nonprofit basis, and like a health maintenance organization, would provide care to a set of subscribers who paid for their care through a regular flat fee stabilized by an insurance pool. (The center could also have been pictured as working on a fee-for-service basis.) This center would strive to provide high-quality care to patients at substantial financial savings. It distinguishes itself from other health services in providing a focus for commitment to, and experimentation with, environmental principles in health care.

The Green Health Center's code of ethics articulates its commitment to environmental sustainability but does not touch on the details of traditional and conventional professional ethics commitments such as confidentiality and truth-telling. We assume that clinicians will continue to treat patients in an ethical and respectful manner in the GHC just as they now (hopefully) do in traditional institutions. Health care should generally give primacy to its usual goals: to treat the sick, relieve suffering, and foster rehabilitation and functionality where illness cannot be cured (Hanson and Callahan 1999). But a natural result of integrating these traditional goals with environmental responsibility is that priorities among goals may shift and new goals may be added.

Here we present the Working Group's document, "The Green Health Center: Ethical Principles and Purpose," with comment on each of its points. The code or "manifesto" consists of a preamble and twelve guiding principles.

Ethical Principles and Purpose of a Green Health Center

Preamble

Human well-being is dependent on the intact functioning of earth's ecological systems. And the well-being of individuals and families is dependent on access to health care and public health, together with other basic social goods. The Green Health Center (GHC) will provide high-quality health care consistent with ecological sustainability and fairness. The provision of health care for present generations must not undermine the ability of ecosystems to support future generations. Health-care practice must reinforce the restoration and maintenance of global ecosystems. The clinical and environmental activities of health care must be conducted with fairness and without exploitation.

The preamble is intended to echo Herschel Elliott's principle of ecological dependency and also to express the Brundtland definition of *sustainability*, which holds that human health needs to be a long-term concern transcending generations. Not only does the GHC intend to avoid harm to the ecosystem, it strives to be involved in rehabilitating global ecosystems. In treating its individual patients, it metaphorically considers the earth as a patient also: the patient who embraces all patients (Somerville 1995).

Guiding Principles of the Green Health Center

1. The GHC provides health care in ways that minimize harm to human and ecosystem health. In order to avoid harm, two key points must be recognized and integrated into health care. First, the main environmental human-health problems created or exacerbated by the medical system itself must be recognized and measures taken to mitigate them. Second, health professionals, nonclinical health-care workers, and patients need to develop, as an integral part of their conception of patient care, a philosophy of health that respects both human biology and the place of humans in nature.

2. The architecture, organizational design, strategic planning, management, and budget of the GHC embody principles of responsibility to nature and future generations. The GHC should strive to be environmentally conscious as an integrated whole. Although virtually all hospitals and clinics comply with legal environmental requirements and some, such as Fletcher Allen in Burlington, Vermont, go beyond them to express environmental concerns in a variety of programs, we do not know of any provider that is thoroughgoing in its attention to sustainability (Achtenberg and Grossman 1995).

Sim Van der Ryn and Stuart Cowan open their book *Ecological Design* by saying,

If we are to create a sustainable world—one in which we are accountable to the needs of all future generations and all living creatures—we must recognize that our present forms of agriculture, architecture, engineering, and technology are deeply flawed. To create a sustainable world we must transform these practices. We must infuse the design of products, buildings, and landscapes with a rich and detailed understanding of ecology.

(Van der Ryn and Cowan 1996, ix)

There are many sources for such principles that health care can borrow from and adapt, such as the permaculture, New Alchemy, and deep ecology movements (Mollison 1990; Todd and Todd 1994; see also Alexander 1977; Lyle 1985; McKenzie 1991).

Environmental problems stem partly from ecologically unsound design. If people ignore the connections between the built environment and the planet, we end up destroying nature and our own health. *Ecological design* is defined by Van der Ryn and Cowan as "any form of design that minimizes environmentally destructive impacts by integrating itself with living processes" (Van der Ryn and Cowan 1996, x) (see note 1). One mistake that people make when they think about ecological limits is to expect that our cities and buildings will be less beautiful, less exciting—just *less*. But ecological design holds the promise of a world that is healthy, esthetically rich, comfortable, convenient, and harmonious with nature. Thinking creatively about design—both on a large scale, as in the design of hospital buildings, and on a smaller scale, as in the design of medical products and technologies and their processes of manufacture—is one of the ways the greatest strides toward sustainability in health care can be achieved. Principles of ecological design have been articulated in great detail for particular realms of activity such as farming or water management; similar work is needed to develop coherent ecological design principles for health care.

In February 2002, a working group initiated by the Commonweal Foundation undertook such a creative effort under the title "Ecological Medicine," which the group defines as "a field of inquiry and action to reconcile the care and health of ecosystems, populations, communities, and individuals." The Commonweal group emphasizes the following principles for health care (Myers et al. 2002, quoted and paraphrased):

- *Interdependence*. The health of individuals and the success of medicine rest on the healthiness of populations and communities, and all of these ultimately depend on the health of the earth's ecosystem.
- *Resilience*. Healthy humans and the earth's ecosystems cannot rest in a steady state; they depend on dynamic interactions marked by resilience. Therapy must rest on the ability of humans to recover and heal in an ecological context. Systems that are integrated with—and mimic—the elegance, economy, and resilience of the natural world offer promising paths for health-care techniques (Benyus 1997).
- *Precautionary principle*. The current regime of medical technologies has moved too far from the principle of "do no harm," particularly where harm extends to

the human community and to nature. The precautionary principle is significantly more conservative than current practice with regard to risk-taking and potential harm.

- *Appropriateness.* In its Greek origins, *medicine* means "appropriate measures." Our understanding of what is to be appropriately offered in clinical medicine needs to be readjusted by a better sense of how therapies fit into a larger picture of public health, community, and the burden on earth's ecosystem.
- *Cooperation.* Stronger cooperation is needed among clinicians and ecologists, and health-care organizations need to be managed with more active participation by the communities they serve. To promote welfare and conserve resources, competitiveness should be subordinated to cooperation to promote welfare and conserve resources. Communities should achieve their health and welfare programs within the capacities of their regional ecosystems.
- *Urgency.* This revolution in thinking about health care and society justifies a substantial commitment of social resources without delay.

Architecture, one of the primary areas in which concepts of green design are already being applied, is particularly important, since new and redesigned buildings often mark the inception of new enterprises. Buildings involve substantial resources in their construction and commit institutions to decades (hopefully centuries) of resource flow in maintenance and remodeling. The architectural planning process can educate administration and staff by helping them to imagine new opportunities for applying ecological concepts. A few green buildings have already been constructed for health-care institutions, and architectural firms increasingly include criteria relevant to sustainability in their designs (Wright and Maine 2001).

Some concepts of ecological architectural design include:

- Siting buildings to integrate with the natural flow of air and water in the area;
- Making nature visible to patients through plantings and sight lines (Frumkin 2001);
- Building-in energy efficiency by methods such as installing efficient lighting sources, exploiting natural lighting, turning lights and air conditioning off with occupancy sensors, turning off larger machines when not in use, using less hot water, building well-insulated walls, taking structural advantage of the angle of sunlight, using solar panels, and urging local power companies to invest in solar and wind energy;
- Reducing water demand by installing gray water systems (diverting waste water to irrigation and landscaping), and installing water-saving showers and toilets;
- Using ecological accounting, materials-flow analysis, and life-cycle analysis in choosing materials;
- Using participatory design processes that include clinicians, patients, and environmentalists;
- Remodeling older buildings to conserve resources;

- Protecting local species and fostering urban wildlife habitat on the hospital grounds;
- Establishing good public transit and bicycle connections; using environmentally designed vehicles for transporting patients and materials;
- Using local and natural materials;
- Emphasizing recycled, durable, nontoxic building materials.

Some of what the Working Group recommended for a GHC are what might be called *light-green fixes*, such as turning off lights and using water-saving toilets. As some health centers have already done, the GHC could experiment with re-establishing solaria, organically managed green spaces, pharmaceutical gardens, and cafeteria composting systems. As the changes become a deeper shade of green, they are likely to begin challenging some of our more deeply entrenched clinical practices (Freeman, Pierce, and Dodd 2000). The care of the sick makes special demands on resources and concepts of design, and these need careful consideration as the practical realization of the GHC is worked out. For example, recycling is generally widely accepted as an important design principle, but the higher infectivity of health-care waste material requires a carefully controlled recycling system. Immunologically compromised patients need special protection from common pathogens.

Tastes and styles may need alteration. For example, composting toilets are highly efficient, safe, and unobjectionable—but they are different from what most Americans are used to (Jenkins 1999). When the circularity of waste with productivity has been made clear, it will be the waste of good fertilizer that offends us.

3. The GHC provides ecologically sustainable therapies and products. The responsibility of health-care institutions to use environmentally friendly products is part of the larger obligation of consumers to accept responsibility for determining how products are made and distributed upstream, especially by choosing products that best fulfill environmental criteria. Because hospitals and clinics purchase large quantities of materials and have personnel and committees who can evaluate products, they are in a better position than individuals to be knowledgeable and influential in their purchasing. In sending out bids for purchasing contracts, for example, hospitals can include criteria for maximizing post-consumer recycled content in supplies, minimizing packaging, and providing for pickup and recycling of waste stream materials.

Ideally, the GHC will conduct a full life-cycle analysis, or similarly complete environmental assessment, on everything it uses, but since many health-care products are complex, ascertaining which supplies or technologies best meet environmental criteria will be a challenging and expensive task. The GHC will have to work on the clearest cases first, make judgements about families of similar products, and establish priorities and rules of thumb for making decisions.

The GHC could join with other hospitals and purchasing consortia in promoting a green labeling program for health-care products. This group effort would work with manufacturers and group purchasing organizations to identify products that are more environmentally sound and label those that meet criteria established by the group. The EPA's Energy Star program, which identifies energy-efficient products such as computers, washing machines, and refrigerators, is a successful example of such a labeling project. Health-care organizations, being relatively few, and tending to work in large, powerful purchasing groups, could potentially put green labeling programs to effective use.

The GHC might consider the following criteria for green purchasing:

- Buy locally when possible. In general, supplies made locally will involve less impact because transportation costs are reduced.
- Use renewable sources.
- Substitute greener products for environmentally more-harmful products. For example, just as hospital pharmacies substitute less-expensive drugs for more-expensive prescriptions, a list of greener drug substitutions could be kept as well.
- Use simpler items. The simpler an item, the less energy, transportation, and tools are likely to be involved in its production.
- Reuse. Although the capital costs of cleaning and reprocessing durable materials and equipment are high, the persistent dumping of products into landfill ultimately produces high volumes of waste. Most environmentalists view reusables as superior, although the difference between the two is sometimes marginal. Case-by-case analysis is needed.
- Reduce toxicity. Cases of egregious toxicity were discussed in Chapter 4, such as mercury and dioxins. Some medications, however, do their work by being toxic or are toxic at high doses (see note 2). There are medications so toxic to the environment even in small amounts (such as some radiological materials) that the GHC might refuse to use them. For other medications, clean manufacture and disposal may be the key. As patients, we need to be responsible about what flows through our bodies, and more engaged in the environmentally responsible disposal of both prescription and over-the-counter medications.
- Use less. The technological difficulty of reducing the environmental impact of product manufacture, use, and disposal suggests that modest consumption is one of the key principles of environmentally sound health care. This principle, of course, has to be balanced with good patient care.

In addition to reducing the overall size of their waste stream by buying and using resources more carefully, health-care institutions can clearly also treat waste more carefully. They should:

- Discontinue using incinerators and switch to autoclaving or microwaving infectious materials. Perhaps better sterilization processes can be developed.

- Segregate waste. Some of this is already done, but not enough care is taken in keeping ordinary waste out of the red-bag waste stream, which is much more expensive to process. And more fundamentally, items should be designed to simplify segregation of different materials in the product after use.

4. The GHC provides services to patients with any health condition but may limit the range of therapies offered in order to reduce ecological impacts and increase efficiency.   Given the reduction in scale that environmental changes will be pressing upon the First World, it is clear that a sustainable health-care center would have to limit the services it can offer. The obvious place to start is with the least valuable procedures; it has often been suggested that health care would be substantially more efficient if it were to eliminate harmful and ineffective procedures and conduct fewer diagnostic tests. This reasonable suggestion has proven politically difficult to implement, for there are no procedures without their advocates and dependents, nor are profitable medications necessarily coextensive with safe and effective ones. The GHC might provide a politically more realistic and effective model by which to make progress toward this objective, because its break with traditional practice would be strong and clear, and its rationale for cutting costs would rest on the deep foundation of ecological sustainability.

But since a sustainable health-care service will have to be scaled down by half or more compared to current practice, it is likely that a number of effective and desirable services will need to be utilized only minimally or eliminated altogether. This is a more daunting prospect. When one member of the Working Group presented the idea of the GHC to a bioethicist, he angrily responded, "What a perfect way to eliminate undesirable patients!"

In fact, individuals who are usually regarded as "less desirable" from the perspective of industrialized acute care may be better served by medicine from an environmental perspective. Putatively undesirable patients are typically those with disabilities or those with long and discouraging programs of rehabilitation. To the cost-conscious, such patients arouse concern because the price of their care adds up over the years, reimbursement rates tend to be lower than on technologically oriented acute services, and the care is less interesting to some staff. But since the equipment and technology typically employed by such patients are often relatively simple—wheelchairs, braces, feeding tubes, and the like—they may well be more attractive to the GHC. What such patients often need is considerable human assistance, and it is our assumption that human labor is nowhere near as costly to the environment as technology. And costs spread out over time are more easily sustained.

Difficult unresolved questions of how to set limits remain. If the GHC were to minimize the availability of ventilators, would we then have to employ Intensive Care Unit selection criteria so strict that we unintentionally discriminated against the most vulnerable patients? What simpler or palliative therapies would we offer to patients that would be preferable to more intensive therapy? What should be said to help the healthy GHC subscriber who buys in because he or she expects to stay healthy in the near future, but who suddenly finds himself or herself unexpectedly in a desperate condition for which environmentally extravagant options exist?

A partial answer to these questions of setting limits is that joining the GHC is voluntary. Since the Green Health Center competes as one enterprise among many providers offering health care to the public, voluntariness and autonomy could stand as partial protection for the ethics of limits. The GHC needs to have strong blue-sky contractual requirements, so that patients are clearly informed of what services are excluded. Moreover, representative groups of patients need to participate in planning the extent of services to be offered. Patients then can ethically be told "no" with regard to therapies the GHC does not provide (Daniels 1986). Patients who want more will be referred to more-traditional services at their own or their insurer's cost. Such practices differ little from the myriad situations now when patients run out of benefits or face contractual managed-care limitations.

There are many ways to set limits, and a range of possible methods can be considered. For example, instead of eliminating Intensive Care Units altogether, resource use can be limited by restricting the number of beds in the units and by using strict admissions criteria (Yeaworth 1997). The Working Group assumed that the GHC would offer certain therapies, and that clinicians would be able to allocate these as needed without thinking about limits. The idea is to strive, while respecting limits, to restore a feeling of abundance. Although they will be involved in setting the GHC's general resource policies, clinicians can devote a full measure of care without making harsh individual resource decisions at the bedside.

In limiting the range of therapies it offers, the GHC proposes to do what some philosophers would call rationing. The term *rationing* has a number of common uses, and what the GHC proposes is like rationing in some respects, but *rationing* is not the right term for practices proposed here. "Rationing" is usually used in bioethics to refer to practices that conserve resources by providing patients with "less than optimal" care (Ubel 2000). But, the notion of *optimal* needs a context: If resources are never to be considered, then the concept of "optimal" care is completely wide-open and without limit: in fact, a fantasy. *Optimal* needs to be understood as "optimal within the resources available," or "sustainable optimal care." What passes for optimal care at the larger medical centers, because it is so extraordinarily expensive, is wasteful, intemperate, and ultimately ecologically destructive.

Our hope is that a more modest package of services will be attractive to most people, who may be willing to trade off less involvement in health care, less risky courses of therapy, and less elaborate rescues in order to spend more of their lives free of involvement in health care and free of the burdens of working to pay for it.

While the GHC struggles with the questions of what therapies to omit, it can also design and build a package of positive and valued services oriented more to an ecological and environmental sense of health and disease. It will, for example:

- Emphasize reproductive and family planning services that educate patients about issues of population size and growth;
- Emphasize patient education toward healthy living—the GHC would actually do what managed-care institutions promised to do;
- Provide resource-conservative therapies that contribute to healthy lives, such as massage, yoga classes, exercise programs, healthy-cooking lessons, and counseling;
- Build palliative care services;
- Participate actively in neighborhood-based planning for weather disasters, food shortages, economic disruptions, and other likely twenty-first century events, including interruptions of health-care supplies and materials;
- Build nearby voluntary mutual and community care services that can provide a strong element of help during therapy and recovery;
- Adopt a balanced approach to infections, neither neglecting their power nor overusing dangerous counteragents;
- Use the more effective and comforting of complementary and alternative medications, but subject them to the same standards of efficacy, danger, and life-cycle environmental cost as allopathic medications;
- Encourage longer visits between patients and health professionals and more hands-on personal care;
- Make home visits to survey environmental problems and to assist in remedying problems at home, such as helping people clear out their medical chests, identify sources of lead, and dispose of old pesticides;
- Limit heroic end-of-life services.

5. The GHC engages in a continuous process of assessment and evaluation of its services, in light of both patient satisfaction and research into environmentally preferable technologies. Ongoing evaluation and research into the environmental aspects of GHC services must be an important component of its activities. Since the environment is changing rapidly, what counts as environmentally sound technology will keep changing. Equipment and processes change quickly and are so complex that we often must guess the consequences of our actions, or use information-conservative principles like the precautionary principle.

Consistent with its environmental commitment and small scale, the GHC will balance the collection of information with the environmental and financial costs of acquiring it. So, while it will make use of information technology, it will continue to rely primarily on fostering observant, alert, outspoken staff and on continuing input from patients and the community.

Although some may worry that a lean package of health-care services might lower the overall quality of care and increase poor outcomes, the present high rates of error in traditional medicine, with a mortality rate on the order of the automobile mortality rate in the United States, suggest that environmentally sound health care might be made much safer than health care on the industrial model (Kohn, Corrigan, and Donaldson 2000).

6. The GHC employs ecologically sound conceptions of health, recovery, and rehabilitation. Ecologically sound philosophies of medicine and health proved to be one of the more controversial topics of the Working Group. When the Working Group began its discussions, our attention was largely focused on limiting allopathic medicine as it is ordinarily practiced, but even the briefest discussion of the Green Health Center with interested members of the public excited support from those enthusiastic about the wellness movement and naturopathic healing methods. We were at first reluctant to go this route, since so many alternative health measures are unevaluated, and if a host of untested dietary supplements and herbal therapies were added to the allopathic pharmacopoeia, we would only increase the environmental impact of health care.

But this public point of view contains wisdom. If treatment were only to return patients to consumerist lifestyles, then the Green Health Center would fail to serve its general purpose of reducing the environmental impact of a healthy life. Naturopathy and similar philosophies teach that people should learn to live in more natural ways. A return to "normal" health involves a return to an ecologically sounder lifestyle. Insofar as methods are found to be "natural" and modest in resource consumption, and safe and effective, they should generally displace risky allopathic methods based ultimately on fossil fuel precursors.

Commonplace or commercially generated conceptions of "natural" medicine seldom withstand rigorous examination (Callahan 1996; Callahan 1998, 125–129; McGee 1997, 52–55; Saito 2002), but they express important ideals many people adhere to. If developed carefully, concepts like "natural" and "organic" might be useful in distinguishing sustainable from unsustainable therapies and products. Thus, the Working Group considers it a useful project of the GHC to reconcile conceptions of *nature* used in environmental protection with those commonly applied to health and consumer goods.

Health care should discourage patient dependency on medicine, encourage healthy lifestyles, prefer attentive staff to technology, and eliminate unnecessary treatment. Corporate health care, investing heavily in technology and bureaucracy while paying less attention to employees and their relationships with patients, tends increasingly to contradict its own ideals and fails to respond to self-criticism.

The ecology of the human body needs more consideration. An extensive literature exists in this area, from which the designers of the GHC can learn, beginning with René Dubos' great work on human adaptation and disease (Dubos 1965; 1966;

1968; Dubos and Escande 1980). For example, disease-generating viruses, bacteria, and fungi are typically regarded as an "axis of evil" in health care. Too many public health programs intended to eradicate major diseases have met with failure; containment and mitigation have usually been more realistic goals (Siddiqi 1995). Modern medicines, together with the massive deployment of antibiotics in meat, are stimulating bacterial evolution at rates already dangerous for humans (Schmidt 2002).

It is possible that some minor infections will go untreated at the GHC, since for most people they are self-limiting; while other widespread infections, on the model of invasive species, may receive a higher priority than they now would be given. For instance, a green system of health care would take much more seriously the diseases associated with poverty—malaria, HIV/AIDS, and tuberculosis—and their expectable spread in the United States. The GHC would be active in programs to improve the health of the poor, such as support for good nutrition and educational campaigns about needle use and the spread of AIDS.

7. The GHC encourages staff and patients to live in environmentally sound ways that express a modest level of consumption.   Patients and staff of the GHC have responsibilities to maintain healthy and modest lifestyles. Given the nature of the enterprise, the GHC is likely to attract people committed to environmental values, so our work will already be partly done. The GHC would maintain an active program of assistance and education to help patients reduce consumption, and it would work with the patients to promote ways of life that are more respectful of nature, such as

- Promoting vegetarianism;
- Joining public campaigns against harmful products such as junk food, alcohol, drugs, tobacco, guns, and automobiles;
- Supporting community efforts to reduce consumption;
- Promoting communitarian approaches to health; and
- Recognizing that healing the earth is part of health care.

What should be done, if anything, when patients continue to lead unhealthy lives? Working Group members considered it unfeasible, inhumane, and a violation of privacy to discriminate against people who live unhealthy lives by excluding them altogether as patients. Nevertheless, the group agreed that the global situation is urgent enough that the GHC must be active in influencing the lifestyles of its members by educational programs and incentives. In any case, active health education could be lent a stronger atmosphere of autonomy by writing the contract in such a way that subscribers make some behavioral agreements. Proponents felt that strong educational involvement and influence by health practitioners is part of community support, related to the old tradition of making home visits. The concept of the individual as interconnected biologically and chemically with the earth alters traditional conceptions of personal identity; in this context professionals may legitimately concern themselves with how people eat and treat their bodies.

The GHC could use a wide variety of "soft" encouragements with patients: education (green information in the waiting rooms), and modeling environmental values by providing local and organic foods, unbleached toilet paper, and low-wattage lighting, bicycle parking places, and similar measures readily noticeable by patients.

With regular in-service programs and an enlightened architectural ambiance, the center could foster modest and healthy staff lifestyles. It may also be possible to provide programs for staff to live near the Center and to encourage energy-efficient transportation (such as walking) to and from work.

8. The GHC acts as a community educator, advocating principles of sustainability in every aspect of life. The responsibility of the GHC as educator and advocate extends beyond patients and staff to encompass the wider community. The GHC would seek to maintain an educational presence: for example, by offering programs and materials on health and the environment to schools and community groups, perhaps staffed by volunteers from among its older patients. The GHC would be strongly involved in prevention, not just for its own patients but for the whole community. It would take an active role in advocating support for public health infrastructure, such as clean water and air, and safe streets and housing. It would aim to help the community strengthen public-health goals and integrate them with goals for environmental improvements. It should, for example, become involved with programs such as lead testing, bioremediation (using living organisms to degrade toxic contaminants), participation in the United Nations "Healthy Cities" program, and encouraging local urban and town green spaces.

The GHC would actively support sustainable local economic development such as neighboring small businesses involved in clean production, recycling, and organic foods (Rodger 2001). By conducting research on environmentally sound methods of health care, it could encourage the development of new businesses producing greener health-care technologies.

In addition to designing its own buildings sustainably, the GHC should help other local projects include health and environmental values in their architecture. Working openly for community change, it would be much more active politically than traditional health-care institutions. The GHC draws heavily on patients' sense of community responsibility and a willingness of both staff and patients to get off their couches and away from the television long enough to engage in community activity.

9. The GHC encourages institutions with which it has business and academic relations to operate in environmentally responsible ways. A key way for the GHC to promote green practices is to be a good green consumer and educator. It can choose to do business with companies that have strong environmental records, and it can provide education and research that aids other companies in avoiding health and environmental risks.

It can strive to avoid working with companies with poor environmental practices. (This may pose some interesting ethical questions for patient care: what if a company operating unethically provides a useful medication?) It may resist a new mall development by declining to place a branch office there. It should maintain a socially responsible investment portfolio, and in particular avoid investing in companies producing tobacco and other products harmful to human and ecological health (Boyd, Himmelstein, and Woolhandler 1995).

10. The GHC pays its share of the environmental and social costs of providing health care. Many environmental and social costs of economic enterprises are "externalized": unaccounted for in the budgets of corporations. These include such costs as water pollution, global warming, and displaced populations. Although the activities of private enterprises often play a significant role in creating these problems, the costs of cleaning them up are usually borne by taxpayers in general. In contrast, the GHC would strive, along with other responsible corporations, to bring the prevention and amelioration of these consequences into its full budgetary account.

Some of these costs could be addressed by paying into funds for environmental cleanups; in other cases, environmental harm could be balanced by direct remediation projects. The GHC could plant trees to compensate for the paper it uses. Inevitably, this approach will tend to raise the costs of providing health care, but without a true system of accounting for real environmental costs we cannot hope to strike a sustainable balance among ecosystem, population, and individual health.

Could the GHC be economically viable in the current economic environment? Perhaps. It would probably function best as a not-for-profit organization, possibly a cooperative. The GHC would probably be a good long-term investment, since it is designed to be more durable, with low costs and modest capital, than the present oversized health service system. As larger systems break down, the smaller, better designed GHCs may be able to compete effectively against institutions with larger capital commitments. Accordingly, the success of the GHC should not be measured in terms of the productivity of labor, but by measures such as customer and employee satisfaction. Labor costs should be kept low and on a flat, equitable scale. The GHC should be able to make up for low salary scales at the high levels by better job satisfaction derived from the meaningfulness of work, more time with patients, good cooperative working relations, lower costs of living at home, a stronger sense of autonomy, and more satisfactory feelings of acting responsibly.

11. The GHC monitors, minimizes, and equalizes environmental risks to GHC employees. Health care exposes employees to many risks, such as infections, radiation, allergens, and toxic chemicals. In keeping with its general goal to protect the environment, the GHC needs to be mindful of hazards to employees; dangerous procedures should be accompanied by shielding, worker-safe disposal equipment and procedures, and infection control. This concern for environmental safety cannot be focused only on clinical workers. Safe cleaning agents should be used by environmental service employees; hospital air quality should be carefully monitored, particularly in areas where instruments are sterilized or waste is incinerated.

12. The GHC provides high-quality services at a level inexpensive enough that they can be made equally available to all. The Green Health Center is designed as a unique and limited social experiment. If it proves to be successful and popular, a version of the GHC might serve as a model for universally accessible health care. But can the GHC be made universally affordable, when many of its practices may well increase the unit cost of some services? For comparison, consider a typical natural foods or organic grocery store. Here, food is often fresher, safer, and more nutritious than that found at the typical supermarket. But it is usually more expensive. A GHC could be designed similarly: patients would receive a full range of the best and safest health-care services using environmentally sound materials at a significantly higher price. But this would defeat its purpose. In order to make the overall package less costly—in the interests of distributive justice—the pressure on the range of services could be severe. It may turn out that the initial unique green health center may be too expensive to be universally available; if the idea is widely copied, however, the financial costs of environmentally sound production will surely decline.

The Working Group considered offering services that could feasibly be made available worldwide, but the United States is so far from accepting what is needed for global justice that it would be an achievement just to offer health-care services modest enough that they could be extended nationwide. Although it may be tempting to consider a stratified range of Green Health Centers oriented toward what patients of different incomes can afford, both sustainability and justice argue strongly against this concept. As the above principles indicate, the GHC is committed to providing an ample range of services that standard health care does not now provide. If it is to minimize both its environmental impact and its prices while adding these environmentally related services, it will need to keep thinking in terms of simplicity and modesty of scale.

Processes for Allocating Resources

One of the difficult problems in designing the GHC is establishing processes for setting the overall scale of the GHC while establishing priorities for care and eventually making specific decisions about what procedures and materials to use.

The first stage will consist of what architects and designers sometimes call a "visioning" process to give further definition to the vague description of the GHC presented here. With its roots in town planning, the visioning process brings experts and stakeholders together in order to design a complex project such as a building or regional economic plan. By linking formation of the plan with a process involving public members, it can gain legitimacy and involve people as advocates of the project (Ames 1994).

In the first step of the visioning process, participants will work with small groups of experts and with public focus groups to inventory available resources. In the case of the GHC, the limits set by sustainability will be emphasized and interpreted, whereupon more specific criteria can be developed and additional decisions made about products and therapies. Such committees should not be confined to clinicians and administrators; if patients and members of the public play an active role, patient involvement in health-care decisions can move upstream, where patient autonomy can shape the clinical environment more effectively than at the bedside.

There are really two facets to the problem of setting the scale of the GHC. On the environmental side of the equation, priorities are needed for mitigating and eventually turning around environmental degradation. On the clinical side, therapies need to be classified according to their value to patient care, balanced by their environmental impact.

Balancing the Environmental and the Clinical

Setting priorities for environmental concern is inherently ambiguous. Should we be most concerned about energy, toxics, wilderness preservation, creating new technologies, poverty, establishing new rules for economic relationships, or what?

Doubtless, the correct answer is "all of the above." But since the planet is in such a broad environmental crisis, the pursuit of one goal is likely to interfere with the accomplishment of another. Switching energy production from fossil fuels to biomass requires more arable land than may be available, given population pressures. Preserving wilderness may conflict with the needs of the neighboring poor and their harvesting of basic materials for living. Helping people be more in touch with and appreciative of the natural world, as with ecotourism or guided trips into remote wild areas, may put our remaining wilderness at increasing risk.

Those who started the GHC project hoped that they would be able to set ecological priorities. But striking a balance among environmental and health-care goals is a large project that requires a legitimate, formal, and creative visioning process involving a wide range of interested and knowledgeable people. There will be so many uncertainties in the next decades about what sudden events and new technologies may reshape our perception of our health and environment that the general choice of level of activity for the GHC must involve carefully thought-out guesswork. Here are four alternate formulations that use different ways to set goals:

1. The visioning project would define the scale and design of the GHC with reference to the four elements of health constituting ecological medicine: environment, public health, community, and health care. This goal seems to bite off much more than such a small institution can possibly chew, since the main factors in maintaining human health are in the practices and economic infrastructure of society in general, not health care in particular. The main efforts for human health cannot take place in medicine. Instead, the GHC should address the specific technological and personal needs that can, without excessive environmental expense, supplement ecosystem, community, and public health. But a reasonable guess as to appropriate relative expenditures of resources in each of the four areas could be used to shape some of the GHC's local priorities.
2. Envisioning the GHC might be guided by a rough calculation of a *sustainable* per capita ecological footprint of health care; that is, the approximate area of land needed to maintain the activities of health care for each person (Germain 2001–2002). The calculation would take into account health care's "fair share" of reductions compared with other realms of social activity. This process could focus on the factors controllable at levels of purchase, use, and disposal.
3. Another approach would consider a "basic minimum" or "decent minimum" for health services, and would then strive to provide that level of care in as green and sustainable fashion as possible.
4. Visioning might also classify therapies and products into different types and estimate their environmental cost versus their clinical benefit. They could then be ordered by ratio from the most beneficial at least environmental cost to the least beneficial at most cost. The GHC would then simply buy as many of the most valuable and least costly therapies as it could afford.

Other approaches are possible. What is important is that the decision be the result of a careful collective judgement and be formulated in a clear enough fashion that criteria for assessing health care practices and products can be defined, prioritized, and communicated to prospective participants.

The Oregon Plan

The GHC can be seen as representing a green version of the "Oregon Plan," a noted public effort to limit costs by a democratic and open process. The Oregon Plan established a mixed professional and public process by which to determine a selection of services to be made available to Medicaid patients in order to extend coverage to all in Oregon who were medically indigent and many who were nearly so. Consistent with this level of coverage, the intention was to maintain a plan to provide the most needed services within the capacity of the public budget. The concept is simple: public focus groups first engaged in a dialogue over what they valued in health care, such as care for the aging, safety, recovery of function, emergency care, and so on. Health professionals then rated about 700 major treatments in reference to these values. The plan thus used a conceptual division common in health care between values on the public side and objective information on the professional side. The Oregon legislature authorized the Medicaid program to cover the highest-rated items (Bodenheimer 1997a, 1997b; Mehlman 1991; Strosberg et al. 1992).

Although there is some disagreement among observers, the Oregon Plan has been particularly successful in meeting its goals of setting priorities, reducing costs, and allowing publicly funded care to be more widely accessible. It has certain weaknesses for our purposes, however: The Oregon Plan did not do a cost-benefit analysis of therapies; it only listed therapies according to their value—not their effectiveness. For example, treatment of coma, an often futile procedure, was at one point the highest priority on the list of therapies. It is possible that if likelihood of success and the environmental cost of therapies were also included, a more valuable set of therapies could be found while minimizing environmental cost.

Since the Oregon Plan was concerned with financial and not environmental costs, the cost side of the equation was analyzable in relatively simple, single-valued terms (dollars). But environmental consequences vary; so for green purposes, therapies will need to be classified by *type* of environmental cost as well as *degree*. Last, and perhaps most important, the plan had some people thinking about how to set limits for other people: the priorities were set through a wide public process, but were designed for care to be received only by the poorest members of the public, who composed only a minority of public members involved. In contrast, the abnegation involved in the Green Health Center would hopefully involve patients and clinicians in thinking of their own and their families' lives and health.

Conclusion

Our aim in this chapter has been to reflect on the application of environmental considerations to the health-care setting: whether it is ethically possible, and what a thoroughly ecological perspective on health care sounds like to our ears. The GHC Working Group's thought experiment resulted in a mission statement and principles that we believe to be worthy of serious reflection. Although there is a sensible concern that health-care services responsive to the environmental crisis might involve patients' and caregivers' excessive abnegation, most of the GHC makes sense to many people and would provide widely acceptable services. Green health services appear, then, to be morally feasible, if we take "moral feasibility" to mean that they:

- Meet important obligations and expresses a sense of responsibility;
- Can be designed without violating important moral obligations;
- Are possible.

There might well be controversy on this last point. Some who have read the GHC Working Group's mission statement charge it with being "too idealistic." These critics seem in fact to mean "unrealistic" or "impractical": the idea is economically impossible. But if the enterprise makes sense ethically, offers something of value, and is realistic in considering long-term environmental needs, there may be ways to work out the flow of salaries, fees, and investments, even in a larger economic environment that is unfriendly to ecological concerns.

Existing health-care institutions cannot easily halve themselves in one fell swoop, but they could set themselves the modest and easily attainable goal of the immediate reduction by 10% of their environmental burden. Many changes involve simple fixes or shifts in daily habits, and integrating them should raise no particular moral concerns. An extensive literature exists on green design, eco-efficiency, dematerialization, and green purchasing in industry; the knowledge and many of the technologies are already on the shelf.

Unfortunately, American bioethics seems generally to give little attention to the global predicament facing industrial medicine in the next half century, and by and large accepts medical materials, science, and techniques as given. Yet the trends and aims of modern American medicine are incompatible with an ecological approach to the global situation, committed as it is to central corporate ownership, complex global sources of supply, the exploitation of nature, high toxicity, and fossil fuels. In contrast, the philosophy of ecological design is one of decentralization, regionalization, nontoxicity, and renewable resources. Bioethicists need to develop a stronger sensitivity to these options.

Notes for Chapter 5

1. Five Principles of Ecological Design (from Van der Ryn and Cowan 1996)

"Solutions grow from place." Design should begin from an intimate knowledge of place, should be small-scale, and should respond to local conditions and needs.

"Make nature visible." Making the processes of nature visible within design can help keep us informed of, and in tune with, our place in nature.

"Design with nature." Design should work with natural processes of regeneration; for example, by creating systems that reprocess their own waste or by combining two systems, where the waste from one provides the fuel for the other.

"Ecological accounting informs design." Information about environmental impacts will help shape sustainable design possibilities.

"Everyone is a designer." The design process should be participatory.

2. What Is a Poison?

A poison is any substance that does harm to a body. During the sixteenth century, the Swiss physician Paracelsus first described many components of the modern field of toxicology, including the notion that "The right dose differentiates a poison from a remedy." In the nineteenth century, the Spanish physician Bonaventura Orfila designed systematic methods for testing tissues for toxins for use as legal evidence of poisoning in the French court and investigated the effects of toxins on animals. The growth of the field of toxicology in recent years parallels that of the development of the chemical industry. Pesticides, pharmaceuticals, preservatives, plastics, and sources of energy all have toxicological implications, many unintended and separate from the molecule's purpose.

While all substances are toxic at some level of exposure, they are not equally toxic. Something extremely toxic, like dioxin, will produce death in half of treated animals (LD50) at a microgram dose. Nontoxic substances will cause death in half of treated animals in a much higher dose. Death, however, is not the only toxic effect. Effects can be acute or chronic, reversible or irreversible. They may affect the whole body or be organ-specific. Individuals vary in their susceptibility to toxins depending on species, genetics, gender, age, health, environment, and other factors. Mixtures of substances may lead to complicated effects.

As the number of chemicals produced has grown, so has the need for regulation to protect human and environmental health. In the United States, regulatory agencies include the Food and Drug Administration, the Environmental Protection Agency, and the Occupational Safety and Health Administration. Regulations aimed at reducing risk to human and environmental health reflect Paracelsus' sixteenth-century notion that dose determines whether a substance is a poison or a remedy. Risk depends on hazard (an intrinsic quality of a molecule resulting in toxicity or other damage) and exposure (or dose) according to the equation: risk = hazard x exposure. Genotoxic carcinogens are an exception to this approach. One molecule may be enough to cause cancer, so there is no minimum acceptable dose. Endocrine disruptors, some of which may cause greater physiological effect at a lower dose, may be another exception.

In the past 150 years, risk has been minimized by controlling exposure. Regulations controlling exposure have increased from 25 in 1870 to over 100 in 2000. Protection from exposure at the source does not mean protection from exposure downstream, however. So while regulations may protect those in direct contact with the substance, they do not extend to protect the environment at large. Researchers are now trying to design molecules that minimize unintended toxicity in the first place. Methods for doing this include using computers to test in advance how toxic molecules of a certain shape and composition are likely to be. In this way, populations do not have to depend on physical barriers to reduce their risk of exposure to toxins (prepared by Rachel A. Jameton from Anastas and Warner 1998; Sikdar and El-Halwagi 2001; and Niesink, de Vries, and Hollinger 1996).

3. The Natural Step Priorities

The "Natural Step" is a useful and brief statement of environmental priorities written around 1989 by a Swedish oncologist, Karl-Henrik Robèrt, with the assistance of a physicist, John Holmberg. The program includes with its priorities an organization, a program of advocacy, and an emphasis on working with businesses and industries (Natrass and Altomare 1999). To paraphrase their "system conditions," for a society to be sustainable, it must:

- Draw less material from earth's crust. This means that mining and fossil fuel extraction must be greatly reduced. For health care, this means switching gradually to more durable tools and materials that can be cleaned and reprocessed and preferring new equipment and materials made from previously recycled materials.
- Avoid subjecting the natural world to increasing concentrations of substances produced by society. This addresses the twin problems of downstream toxicity and waste volume. Since so many pharmaceuticals are toxic or involve toxic materials in their production, this is of particular importance for health care.

- Protect biodiversity. Besides requiring reductions in the scale of human activity, as do the first two principles, this principle addresses the particular problem of rapid extinction of species. This last principle has implications for health care: (a) When choosing sites for hospitals and clinics, care should be taken to prevent harming local environments for species maintenance. Buildings and grounds should be friendly to regional species. (b) Pharmaceuticals should be produced from harvestable materials on a sustainable basis. If rare plant or animal species are needed, both that species and the local biological systems that maintain it should be protected.
- Resources should be used fairly and efficiently to meet human needs. This condition allows humanity to meet the three prior conditions more easily by reducing the amount of material needed to foster health and happiness, while reducing unhealthy envy and sources of conflict. The effort to make health care universally available is a part of this project, but so are additional and diverse considerations, such as establishing more equitable salaries among health care specialties and emphasizing the health benefits of equality.

6

At the Bedside

One of the major problems of environmentalism is that its large concern for the fate of the earth seems to overwhelm concern for individual humans. The problems of those who are terminally ill, or facing an unexpected pregnancy or cancer, have an appeal and poignancy for most people that the hard statistics of global decline lack. What medical ethics discussion usually tries to do is to make connections between the local concerns of patients and clinicians and a general framework so that individuals can make decisions that make sense from a larger perspective.

Bioethics, by putting the concerns of patients and clinicians in the larger framework of modern liberal philosophy with its central tenets of individual freedom, scientific objectivity, and social justice, has been building a bridge for the last thirty years between individual cases and a larger conceptual framework. If an ecological framework is to play a more prominent role in bedside bioethics, it will need to supplement the dialogue among clinicians, patients, and ethicists regarding how patient care is conducted.

Who Decides?

A nurse familiar with some of the environmental risks of health care has a young son who is undergoing a surgical procedure in an academic medical center. She is particularly concerned about possible risks to her son from his exposure to PVC (polyvinyl chloride) and DEHP (di-ethylhexyl-phthalate) in plastic bags and tubing used to deliver intravenous medications. She asks that glass and/or other plastics be substituted. Although this is an unusual request, the staff manages to provide equipment composed of alternative materials.

(Hollie Shaner, personal communication)

This story shares much with the garden-variety cases that might be discussed at a medical ethics committee meeting. The patient's choice differs from usual clinical practices and poses some challenges to staff, but it is the kind of choice that most on the ethics committee would agree should be accommodated if possible. An ethicist might argue that the patient's wishes represent a strongly held belief, and draw an analogy with religious principles such as the refusal by Jehovah's Witnesses to accept blood; he or she might advise that staff strive to accommodate patients where they can, even if the staff disagree with the patient's point of view.

Consider an alternative case, in which a patient requests that environmentally sound materials be used, not out of concern for his or her own or family's health, but out of a sense of duty to protect the environment. For example, a patient might prefer that reusable cloth drapes be used in surgery, rather than disposable paper ones. In such a case, the staff may feel that the patient is stepping into an area properly under the hospital's control. Materials management is already complex enough; hospitals cannot easily or efficiently respond to every person's request for special treatment, especially where it does not affect personal interests. The ethics committee may well agree with management: the ethical choice is to respect usual practice.

Yet the cases have more in common than not: environmental concerns should be considered more widely in hospital practices, and should not simply arise as non-standard practices. And although one case involves the patient's interests and the other the patient's duty, they share common ethical roots.

Indeed, the concept of choice is very much at home with actions taken out of regard for others. The doctrine of respect for autonomy is often translated clinically into "respect for the patient's wishes," as though all choice had to arise from self-regarding desires or interests. But dutiful choices can also be made freely; indeed, as we shall discuss more fully in Chapter 8, Kant's initial conception of autonomy was directed almost entirely to expressions of respect for one's duties. The Kantian framework does not regard setting limits on oneself as a loss to one's dignity. In contrast, choice as an expression of desire or wish is a much more modern and consumerist conception.

Nevertheless, decisions about materials should generally be institutional decisions. There are a number of reasons for this. Sometimes environmental improvements are obvious, affect patient care only slightly, and deciding about them would simply overburden patients and clinicians with distracting decisions. At other times, the environmental costs and benefits of materials are uncertain or obscure, and so communication about them could add an overwhelming layer of new complications.

Even so, it may be possible to translate more complex environmental concerns into simpler form for readier communication. One of the achievements of the bioethics movement has been to urge physicians and researchers to translate complex medical matters into language and concepts that patients can understand. If the agenda of bioethics were to make environmental issues a matter of personal choice by patients, then much work would be needed to find new ways to express environmental concerns in immediately understandable language.

The translation problem is only one reason we do not think that conventional bioethics is the right way to handle environmental aspects of health care. The more fundamental reason is that the material foundations of health and health care are, ultimately, socially shared concerns about which decisions should best be made at institutional and community levels.

Institutional Choices

Just like conventional hospitals do, an environmentally oriented institution would establish a background of material standards for patients and clinicians. To some, such a green health care center may seem at first to "disempower" patients because it provides a more modest range of services. Disempowerment, however, would not necessarily be the experience of patients in an environmentally sound hospital. The measure of choice is not the *number* of choices, but the *meaningfulness* of choices, and an environmentally sensitive hospital permits more meaningful choices. By taking global resources into account, the institution allows clinicians and patients to make choices that are more realistic, and thus more significant, in respecting our place in the world. In some ways a modest institution allows a doctor to be more generous in responding to patients: where resources are limited by decision processes away from the bedside, he or she can respond generously to patient needs with what is available.

The costs of health care have risen in recent decades, the severity of illness in the hospital has increased, staffing has been reduced, and the time patients spend with clinicians has shrunk. Patients perceive their choices and control are decreasing, despite efforts to empower them through ethics and the law. Besides permitting more meaningful choices, a green hospital would also enable patients to make morally significant choices by including more public members, representing various patient constituencies, in higher-level planning and decision-making committees. Although systems of public input into institutional administration are difficult to manage, they are worth the effort when the public can influence the organization. Since the design of an environmentally sound health-care institution is a new project and will require many iterations, the public is much more likely to experience a sense of participation than it does with existing institutions.

Meaningful choice could also be enhanced by adding an environmental dimension into the set of considerations affecting an individual's care (see note 1). Different features of the environment are important to different people: some patients may be more concerned about keeping care simple and inexpensive, others may be more concerned with toxicity, renewability, alternative therapies, or the treatment of animals in research. And there are points where opening the bedside to environmental information-sharing and decision-making is particularly appropriate—where patients can safely express their values and where alternative choices will not radically affect the health outcome:

- At discharge. Environmental considerations could be discussed if patients are going to use medications, bandages, or other materials at home during recovery.
- With patients who are neither very sick nor stressed. Such patients are likely to be in a better position to consider the more distant consequences of their care.
- With patients undergoing elective procedures. Patients could consider some of these issues before the procedure is scheduled.
- With environmentally concerned patients. If the health professional knows ahead of time that the patient has environmental sympathies, then such questions are particularly appropriate.

Life, Death, and Environmentalism

Should environmental considerations also come into play when patients are suffering or near death? Many people, both sick and well, have been disappointed by the inhumane aspects of costly high-tech health care and would prefer to follow a simpler path. The countless tales in bioethics of patients who feel coerced and deceived into accepting intensive, costly end-of-life care, and the continuing observations by nurses of excessive life-saving efforts in some university hospitals, testify to the desire for simpler technological approaches, especially to terminal care. We should become better at limiting the costs of dying for those interested in such limits. Patients with serious chronic problems may also be interested in low-key, labor-intensive management of their problems.

In *The Patient as a Person*, Paul Ramsey argued that each human life has incalculable value (Ramsey 1970). It would seem at first glance that a belief in the sanctity of life would lead one to a hasty rejection of environmentalism in medicine. Paul Carrick, for example, argues that deep green principles would necessarily overwhelm the individual, and that the sanctity of life requires that the dying patient be insulated from larger environmental concerns (Carrick 1999). But, as Ramsey noted, choosing to care for a patient without necessarily trying to cure is not a rejection of the sanctity of life. Indeed, to care for the dying, to be fully engaged with that person throughout the dying process, is a strong affirmation of life—stronger, perhaps, than shutting the patient into an intensive care ward and burying the process of dying under tubes and wires. The concept of *full engagement* harmonizes well with the idea of *interconnection* among people and nature so characteristic of environmental philosophy. And the truth is, patients often want less than is offered and become involved in quixotic treatment near the end of life as a result of institutional and professional momentum, not their own desires and values.

Bioethics has made a contribution to professionals' and patients' ability to discuss death openly. This openness provides an opportunity near death for patients, their families, and caregivers to engage in thoughtful conversations on the use of technology in keeping people alive, and on balancing an individual's claim on life against the use of resources for other purposes. Rather than hindering such discussions, an environmental perspective would add depth to these considerations. When one appeals to such ethical considerations, abstract images and ideas come into play that not only affect decisions but also allow a consideration of the inevitability of death, our commonality with other creatures, and its healthy place in the environment (see note 2).

The fears expressed—often by older people—not so much of death, but of attempts to rescue them from death, are understandable given the unnaturalness of the hospital. Many people feel sustained, or at least comforted, by their exposure to nature; the home's primacy as a site of hospice care arises partly from its closeness to the garden, a view of the yard, and the birds, dogs, cats, rabbits, or people that pass by. The hospital often moves patients away from the comforts and hazards of nature. Part of what is terrifying about the intensive care unit is its bright lighting, the overbearing presence of machinery, its insulation from the outdoors, and the sound pollution of the electronic alarms and overhead announcements. Often a television looms over the bed (death by advertising!). Perhaps the traditional get-well gift of flowers and plants is an effort to bring nature back into the hospital.

What about choosing for others? What about parents who want "everything to be done" for their child? The key to a greener approach will be to create a system in which people can provide their loved ones the best possible treatment, where "best possible treatment" is consistent with equal access for everyone at a sustainable level. Then parents will not be put in a position of having to "deny" care for their children. There will still, of course, be many hard choices to make about whether or not to treat. But one of the problems with our current system is that we never feel we have done enough because no limits are felt to exist in what can be done for a patient.

A troubling case for health professionals is the dying patient who demands treatment that the health-care team considers inappropriate, wasteful, or futile. Often, it is not the patient himself or herself, but a family member or proxy who makes these demands. Within a sustainable health-care system, such problems would arise with less frequency, because the range of services offered would be much smaller— "doing everything you can," based on firm prior agreements, would encompass fewer technological interventions.

The use of advance directives makes good sense from a green perspective, because it can help avoid misapplication of resources. It would seem that we should readily agree with the right of all patients to refuse care. After all, this clearly offers resource conservation. But, as many have noted before, we should not abandon those who refuse care. Some refusals may be based on an unreasonable fear of being burdensome; some may express suicidal depression. In these and other situations, humane intervention may be a much more ethical response than acquiescence to patient demand.

One of the most common immediate reactions to the green health center idea is to suppose that it must certainly include an aggressive campaign for euthanasia—with "End It Fast!" flyers in the waiting rooms—as an obvious route to resource conservation at the end of life. A sustainable health perspective would neither promote nor reject, on principle, physician-assisted suicide or euthanasia. There would be no reason to refuse a patient's request for aid in achieving a meaningful, "chosen" death. On the other hand, were end-of-life care more modest technologically and more robust in terms of humane attention and care, fewer might feel the need to secure a predictable final exit.

Ethics discussion tends to speak of death abstractly and formally, as though it represents a rational choice: death with dignity, the right to die, death decisions, futile therapy, the right to refuse therapy, extraordinary means, and so on. But awareness of death as a natural, inevitable biological process is increasing, as reflected in Sherwin Nuland's moving and detailed descriptions of dying processes (Nuland 1994). Although an individual's death is natural and inevitable, and as such, relatively insignificant on the scale of global evolution, attention and care given to a dying person help maintain community and assert the value of the dying person. There is nothing in the discussion of environmental concern to suggest that respect and attention to these patients should or would thereby be diminished.

Ecological Responsibilities of Health-Care Practitioners

As we discussed in Chapter 4, professional codes, when they refer to environmental responsibilities, often emphasize the role of the professional in shaping organizational choices. No ethical obstacles exist to clinicians' bringing green concepts to the attention of hospital committees involved in planning, budgeting, technology assessment, and other processes that affect the flow of resources. Green clinicians ethically can and should encourage hospitals to be more aware of environmentally related diseases, participate in monitoring health conditions related to global change, and recognize their own contribution to local and global environmental degradation.

The stickier ethical problems arise at the bedside. How strongly should these professional commitments to ameliorate the environmental effects of care influence the actual clinical encounter? Is it ethical, for example, to be concerned at the bedside with the larger framework of resource conservation? Although there are delicate issues involved in bringing environmental concepts to bear on patient care, clinicians can and should be thinking and talking about these issues with patients—perhaps deciding to pursue one form of treatment rather than another, based on environmental considerations balanced with the needs of the patient.

Stewardship

The right balance of global and individual concern is best struck by considering the stewardship model of responsibility. This model arose from theological writing on the relationship between humans and nature. It articulates the biblical injunction to be careful stewards of God's creation. Because of its wide appeal, *stewardship* has become one of the commonest terms denoting environmental responsibility. The notion of clinicians as stewards of resources is not new—indeed, the stewardship model appears in the medical literature with some regularity (though rarely, it must be said, with an eye toward *environmental* conservation). We know that it is part of sound professionalism to consider costs, use materials efficiently, and allocate time and priorities carefully (Jonsen, Siegler, and Winslade 1998). Health-care resources are held in common: the public underwrites medical education and research and serves as experimental subjects; medical knowledge is not "owned" by physicians but held in trust. A similar argument might pertain to drugs, many of which come from natural sources such as plants and minerals, which are also held in common. This view of the "commons" of sustainable health care has much support, and expresses a strong articulation of a stewardship model.

There is a long history of physicians being asked to fulfill social obligations—for example, as advocates of public health through giving immunizations—and voluntarily stepping beyond the confines of their office—as does Physicians for Social Responsibility, which has been active since the 1960s in issues of nuclear deterrence and environmental threats to health.

Stewarding resources with the goal of optimizing what is available to benefit the most people is a legitimate and important obligation that can add richness and depth to the professional's sense of moral responsibility. Critics will quickly point out the dangers of such an expansive notion of professional obligation in health care. Decisions about resource conservation are subjective; they involve decisions about how to value certain human needs or desires against the needs of the community. Yet the accusation of personal bias is not particularly persuasive, since all health-care decisions rely on subjective judgments. And there seem to be legitimate ways to distinguish between value judgments that are benign, such as a physician's intuitive belief in the efficacy of a certain treatment for a certain patient, and those that are pernicious, biased by racial or gender prejudices.

Physicians make resource-use decisions every day. Judgments about medical need and benefit are the natural province of the physician. Yet, allocating services where environmental costs are a consideration would ask physicians to give some weight to environmental values, which they are not yet professionally equipped to do.

Physicians could become more prepared with appropriate information to make more informed and objective decisions as how best to steward resources. A body of information needs to be built that combines data on the efficacy of treatments and their environmental impact. Such an enterprise should follow the model of evidence-based medicine—an attempt to make clinical decisions more scientific and less subjective, and to challenge traditional but unsubstantiated assumptions about best clinical practices. Health-care institutions, materials, environmental services, facilities personnel, professional organizations, and staff bioethicists could help educate health professionals about environmental implications and values affecting their routine resource-use decisions.

One of the main arguments against physicians as stewards for the community is that they would then abandon the patient-centered ethic, a move seen by many in bioethics as dangerous. For example, bioethicist Robert Veatch claims,

Asking a clinician to take on resource allocation tasks is in effect asking him or her to remove the Hippocratic Oath . . . from the waiting room wall and replace it with a sign that reads: "Warning all ye who enter here. I will generally serve your interests, but in the case of marginally beneficial expensive care I will abandon you in order to serve society as their cost-containment agent." (Veatch 2000, 138)

Veatch's wall sign is actually not a bad idea. If physicians are going to take on a stronger role as stewards of resources, it makes sense to be sure everyone understands this, particularly the patient. Instead of this being an automatic point of contention between physician and patient, it is possible to imagine both carefully weighing available options. But physicians can only be put in the role of stewards if it is against a strong backdrop of democratically produced limitations—they cannot be lone rangers of ecological cost-containment. It is better if they work in institutions like the Green Health Center.

Clinicians as Agents of Public Policy

Although clinicians should think of themselves as careful stewards of resources, most of the decision-making about resource use should take place on an institutional level so that clinicians can primarily practice medicine. But there are certain areas where clinicians can actively shape patient behavior, with potentially significant environmental impacts. For example, a nurse or physician might encourage patients to commute to work by bicycle, both because it provides good exercise and because it reduces carbon pollution. Or a physician might encourage patients to eat a vegetarian diet, mainly with the health benefit in mind, but with the additional push toward environmental gains. Are these recommendations overly political? As long as the clinician is focused on the patient's well-being, it is entirely appropriate to encourage both sustainable habits and healthy habits—which, for the most part, overlap (see note 3)

To what extent should environmental concerns about overpopulation shape how a clinician talks to or treats his or her patient? Most factors affecting population arise from social phenomena other than medicine, but population expansion has become one of the key social effects of health care—by increasing longevity, decreasing infant mortality, preventing disease, and successfully treating the seriously injured. It would be obscene, of course, to suggest that health care do its part for the planet by ignoring any of these vital health needs. But there are other ways the goals of health care can and should be made consistent with the goal of reduced fertility: by supporting women's control of reproductive decisions, making safe contraceptives universally available, providing universal access to safe abortion, and by counseling about contraception, infertility, and spacing of children.

It would not be wise to leave providers unguided by policy. Clinicians tend to have their own slant on population issues, and may, for example, be energetic in foisting birth control methods on the poor while catering to the wishes of the wealthy, however little those wishes may serve their clients or the welfare of society. General policies, guidelines, and codes of ethics are useful in the clinical encounter. As it is, professional codes tend to emphasize autonomy in the realm of reproductive choice, which may leave too much room for physicians to let personal attitudes about sex, contraceptives, and abortion shape the clinical encounter. Focused guidance, supported by clear political commitment, is needed; professional codes should give strong support for a broad range of contraceptive counseling and services, including access to abortion.

Health-care professionals have an obligation to support women's choice to have an abortion. Controlling rapid population growth is only one reason. Since contraceptives are of imperfect efficacy, abortion is a necessary adjunct. Access to safe, legal abortion, fundamental to women's health, should be a priority of our health-care system. It is well documented that the ability to space or limit the number of births improves women's health overall.

Matters of Conscience

Health professionals swim in a sea of excess. Although it is tempting, because of the political and relational risks involved, to remain silent about procedures that are environmentally costly and unnecessary, it is important to be clear that the current level of environmental expense and wastefulness of the U.S. health care system is fundamentally morally wrong. It is important to begin the work of cost reduction by being alert to the worst cases. By holding principles different from those in the working environment, the green clinician is rather like an anti-abortion clinician working in a setting that is committed to providing abortions. Important personal commitments must be balanced against the wishes of patients and current policies. Because anti-environmental policies, practices, and beliefs are so pervasive, compromise is usually necessary to preserve such values as community, satisfactory service, and institutional loyalty.

What About the Patient's Responsibilities?

We all have obligations, as potential users of the community's health-care services, to live in ways that promote and maintain our own health and the health of those around us. This is part of a more general obligation to live with a sense of modesty and limits, and with an eye toward respect for nature and for the needs of others. Education will be a vital part of the move toward sustainability. People need to know the basics of a healthy diet: the environmental and health implications of eating meat (including hormones and antibiotics used in animal agriculture), the nutritional deficiencies of fast food, the kinds and quantities of pesticides on fruits and vegetables. We need to understand why exercise is important and why being overweight is a health danger. We need to understand the proper uses of antibiotics and the huge variety of over-the-counter health remedies, so that improper and useless treatments can be kept to a minimum.

These are things patients need to think about outside of the clinic. Is it reasonable also to expect patients to think about environmental responsibilities in the context of their own care? Perhaps. Once in the clinic, patients could remain active by expressing interest in ecological design within health care.

Conclusion

If we stick with the conventional concepts of bioethics, which work well for some aspects of the environmental conversation at the bedside, environmentalism will feel like an intrusion. If we reframe the ethical conversation itself and seek a deeper shift in our understanding of health, health care, and the human relationship to each other and to nature, some of the apparent problems of environmentalism at the bedside will resolve themselves.

Notes for Chapter 6

1. Reusables versus Disposables
   One of the obvious choices that might come up for patients and caregivers is that of reusable versus disposable products. Hospitals use disposable products for just about every need—surgical drapes, bedpans, cups, gowns, gloves, tools, tubes, and IV bags. But aren't disposables environmentally irresponsible? Let us say that one environmentally concerned respiratory care therapist wants to propose to the product-evaluation committee that her hospital switch from disposable to reusable ventilator circuits. She does some research and presents information to the committee. As background, we sketch here some of the basic information about ventilator circuits.

Ventilator circuits are the tubes connecting patients to the ventilator, which helps patients breathe in intensive care units. Each breath provided by the ventilator is artificially heated, humidified, and filtered, just as in the human upper respiratory system. Carbon dioxide and any excess humidity are expelled through the expiratory limb of the ventilator circuit.

Disposable ventilator circuits are made from several different kinds of plastic. Plastics are organic materials using crude oil, natural gas, or agricultural biomass as their basic building blocks. Each kind of plastic imposes its own set of benefits and environmental challenges at every level of production, transportation, use, reuse, and, finally, disposal.

It seemed to our respiratory care therapist that some of the disposable circuits are a poor environmental choice because they are made from PVC, and incineration of PVC can emit dioxins (see note 1, Chapter 4). She would admit that circuits made from PVC have certain advantages such as good shelf-life stability and low cost. But in arguing against disposables, she appeals to the precautionary principle: if dangers exist in a practice, and harm as a result of the practice is difficult to undo, it is best to abstain from the practice, although not all of the data have been compiled.

The respiratory therapist also compared the annual financial costs of reusables with those of disposables. Her estimates showed that, at the time, disposables were only slightly less expensive than reusables. These estimates involved such factors as the purchase price of the tubes, and the costs of their cleaning, storage, and disposal. Despite the small cost difference, then, she concluded that reusable circuits were probably slightly better from an environmental point of view. But she was surprised by how complex obtaining information and making calculations had been. Apparently, the composition of the tubes used at her hospital would change from time to time, as vendors, sources and design changed. And representatives of the companies supplying the tubes often were unsure what a particular model was made of. It was sometimes difficult for those on the products committee to be sure which product was which.

The ventilator circuit case illustrates the kinds of trade-offs that might be considered and the sort of information that is relevant when making decisions about which products to use. The volume and complexity of the information (only sketched here) suggest why most decisions about products and technologies should be made at the institutional level.

Indeed, the complexity of the dilemma of choosing disposable vs. reusable items illustrates a significant principle of environmental savings: *use less*! Perhaps the measure most important in reducing the environmental costs of ventilator circuits turned out to be the decision to change circuits every 48 hours rather than every 24. A clinical study showed that this procedural change apparently did not increase the infection rate. At the same time, the change halved the environmental costs of breathing circuits. There are additional clinical measures by which respiratory therapists might save materials; for instance, by weaning patients faster from the ventilator. Methods include biofeedback and chest physiotherapy, although the environmental costs of these measures must also be taken into account. A research goal should be the development of technologies such as ventilator circuits made from materials that can be cleaned and reused, and that reduce environmental burdens. Nontoxic, energy-conserving cleaning and reprocessing methods need to be developed more widely. In identifying alternative products, we must be careful to assess their life-cycle environmental costs as well.

2. Taxol

Consider a case where concerns for environmental preservation are in tension with the goal of treating serious illness. How would lengthening the lives of patients with cancer balance against the preservation of species?

The drug Taxol, from *Taxus brevifolia*, is one of the success stories of the National Cancer Institute's 1960s screening program that looked for plants, animals, and microbes with anti-cancer properties. Taxol was discovered in 1963, and preclinical work began in 1977 when Taxol was shown to inhibit the replication of human tumor cells. The first clinical trials began in 1983, and in 1992 the Food and Drug Administration approved the use of Taxol in treating refractory ovarian cancer. Taxol is currently used in the treatment of acute leukemia and unresponsive cancers of the ovaries, testes, breast, head, neck, and lung.

Taxol is found in the bark and needles of the Pacific yew, a slow-growing, understory evergreen tree from the family *Taxaceae,* which grows in the virgin rainforests of the Pacific Northwest. The Pacific yew seldom forms pure stands; instead, trees grow haphazardly dispersed throughout the understory. To obtain the bark, the tree must be killed. The five pounds of bark from a typical 200-year-old tree yields only a tiny amount of Taxol: to treat one person with cancer throughout their illness requires the use of approximately six to eight yew trees.

Spurred by the expanded harvest of yew trees and the extinction and destruction of old-growth forests, the Environmental Protection Agency and the Bureau of Land Management issued an environmental impact statement in 1993. As a result, significant resources were allocated to finding alternatives to Taxol. A semi-synthetic form of Taxol, *Taxotere*, has been synthesized from the needles of the European yew tree, which is more abundant than the Pacific yew, and contains a compound more soluble and efficient than Taxol in killing laboratory-grown cancer cells. Although it is FDA-approved, side-effects such as hair loss, mouth sores, and low white-blood-cell counts have reduced its popularity. Another alternative is derived from the needles of the English yew, which contain a compound ten times more concentrated than that found in the Pacific yew. Scientists have discovered, however, that the process of extracting this substance from the tree's needles leaves impurities in the drug.

The majority of Taxol supplied today is a semi-synthetic compound, produced through what is known as the "metal alkoxide process" (MAP). Bristol Meyers Squibb, which has the license over MAP, announced in 1993 that no more bark would be harvested from public lands for the production of Taxol.

Taxol appears to have life-saving benefits for cancer patients, making exclusion of the treatment ethically problematic. Ironically perhaps, the pharmaceutical industry is finding itself allied with environmentalists, since there seems to be a shared interest in preserving the Pacific yew, now listed as a threatened species under the Endangered Species Act. In this particular case, the conflict is gradually being resolved by the development of synthetic alternatives based on fossil fuel precursors. (Prepared by Christina Kerby Kessinger. Sources: National Cancer Institute Cancer Facts 2002; Florida State University 2002; Taxolog Inc. 2000–2001)

3. New Issues for Bioethics

Bioethicists interested in the environmental aspects of health care will find a wide range of ethical issues in need of analysis. The problem of balancing environmental costs with the quality of patient care is expressed in many issues: the use of toxic cleaning agents, whether to open windows at hospitals, the costs of personal choice in a setting committed to modesty, vegetarianism and respect for animals, respect for human life in tension with respect for animal life, the ins and outs of the treatment of obese patients, tensions between conventional and alternative and complementary medicine, and so on. Consideration of facilities and supplies potentially moves bioethicists far from the bedside and from standard concerns with exotic and high-tech materials toward consideration of the relatively ordinary, but just as perplexing and significant, issues regarding supplies, materials, and building techniques seen every day.

In Chapter 5, we supplied an abundance of principles—the importance of place, the visibility of nature, ecological accounting, interdependence, resilience, and so on—which await development, in part through case analyses, in the bioethical arena.

7

Global Bioethics and Justice

When Van Potter first proposed the term *bioethics* in 1970, he described it as the "science of survival." Worried about the unfolding global environmental crisis, he called for a coordinated response from science and the humanities (Potter 1971). By 1990, bioethics had become so strongly associated with the more narrowly focused field of medical ethics that Potter proposed the term *global bioethics* to describe—and encourage—an ethics of health care in the context of global survival and Earth care. A 1995 article cowritten with his daughter Lisa placed global survival on a continuum of acceptability: business as usual would result in a world of "mere" or "miserable" survival where the quality of human existence would be reduced to its lowest levels, largely as a result of excessive consumption and population growth. The Potters envisioned a culture based on global bioethics that would permit an "acceptable" level of survival and a stable state of human health and dignity worldwide. Such a world would be achieved in part by an ethics of restraint in consumption and reproduction (Potter and Potter 1995). In a world of limits, scarcity, and environmental constraints, the morally best world is one in which all people— for many generations—can live with adequate health and quality of life without destroying the ecological basis of species diversity and meaningful community.

Our thinking about health care on a local scale needs to be set within this larger framework. The U.S. health care system reverberates profoundly around the globe. Similarly, what happens around the world has implications for the health of popu-

95

lations in the United States. Our health care and our bioethics have traditionally been quite insular in outlook, and it is important to broaden the view to a global one.

Do We Have Global Responsibilities?

With few exceptions, recent Western moral philosophy has accepted the notion that all humans have moral worth. An obvious implication is that where one happens to live has little bearing on whether or not one has moral standing or is morally deserving of basic human rights and goods. But there is a lively debate in philosophy over whether this means that each person's ethical commitments should be thought of as extending equally to all people, or whether ethics is bounded, with moral commitments arising out of the shared beliefs and local mutual contact among individuals of a particular human community (Booth, Dunne, and Cox 2001; Low 1999).

The latter view, often diagrammed as a series of concentric circles, each disk representing a wider but weaker range of moral concern, derives from the assumption that one's primary responsibilities are to kin and to those nearest geographically, and then weaken as one's connections and relations spread further beyond oneself, concrete connections grow weaker, communication declines, and the mutuality of effects and exchanges lessens.

Although nothing is likely to completely overturn this natural way of looking at responsibilities, environmentalists argue that the balance between central and more peripheral relationships needs to be restruck in some important ways. Most important, of course, is that the rings of responsibility be understood to extend to our *biotic* community (see especially Leopold 1949 and Callicott 2002). More to the point for this chapter, the nature of human and ecosystemic relationships globally is increasing the relevance and moral weight of events and the condition of people at a geographical and political distance.

Environmentalists' vivid sense of global interconnection strengthens this cosmopolitanism in two important ways: all humans must cope with common global circumstances such as climate change, environmental degradation, and the risk of nuclear war; and all humans are strongly interconnected in a global biological community shared with other species and marked by essential flows of material and energy. Human individuals are not seen just as separate entities in voluntary community, but as nodes in a network, inevitably related by global context and material processes. No one is an island.

Global Health

The Concept of Global Health

One cannot read international health documents written over the past few years without noticing the prominence of the phrase *global health*. Bunyavanich and

Walkup, who have reviewed the emergence of the term, suggest that a significant paradigm-shift to global health is occurring, away from the model of *international health*, which is constrained by nation-state boundaries. People, goods, services, pathogens—and prevailing regional levels of healthiness—are increasingly linked on a global scale. For example, the reappearance of malaria in the mid-Atlantic states in the United States is probably related to such cross-border phenomena as immigration, poverty, and climate change (Bunyanavich and Walkup 2001). Addressing local health issues requires a globally coordinated effort.

Professional and academic groups in the United States are recognizing the growing importance of global health. For instance, a 1997 report by the Institute of Medicine called *America's Vital Interest in Global Health* (1997) articulated a concern for global health. The report argues that America has a direct stake in the health of populations around the world, and that American economic, humanitarian, and health interests are best served by active engagement with global health issues, particularly by offering scientific and technological leadership. Echoing the Institute of Medicine report, the Department of Health and Human Services, Office of International and Refugee Health, initiated a new website in 2001 (http://www.globalhealth.gov). The site advises that maintaining the health of Americans requires global concern and that the United States "must engage health policy globally to protect Americans' health and to protect America's vital interests" because increased trade, mass movements of people and goods around the globe, and the growth of international commerce have created new health risks.

Thinking Globally about Disease

As HIV infection rages around the world, health professionals are reminded that humans live in a sea of rapidly adapting microbes and viruses, and that travel and trade make the worldwide spread of infectious diseases inevitable. This appreciation of universal vulnerability represents a renascence of the international health movement that arose after the Second World War, when the World Health Organization was founded to protect travelers from acquiring disease from the regions they visited and to protect regions from the spread of disease by travelers and refugees. The message, then and now, is clear: if a nation or region wishes to be healthy, it must be concerned with infectious diseases around the world and not just at home.

Infectious disease is by many accounts the most serious health condition facing human populations today. It is the leading cause of death, responsible for between a quarter and a third of the 54 million annual deaths worldwide; it accounts for over 40% of the global disease burden, measured in Disability Adjusted Life Years (DALYs). (DALYs measure nonfatal health outcomes. They compare the burden of years lived with a disability or disease with that of premature death, so that mortality does not have to serve as the sole indicator of disease burden.)

The global spread of HIV over the past two decades has been by far the most devastating of the infectious diseases, but the world has also witnessed recent outbreaks of dengue fever (Indonesia), plague (India), cholera (Latin America), and cyclospora (United States), as well as health scares such as Mad Cow disease (United Kingdom). Since 1973, 20 well-known diseases have reemerged and spread, among them tuberculosis, cholera, and malaria. And at least thirty more previously unknown infectious diseases—including HIV, ebola, and Nipah virus— have been identified. The so-called Deadly Seven, responsible for the lion's share of death, are still going strong: HIV/AIDS, tuberculosis, malaria, and hepatitis-B and -C are spreading and in some cases, such as TB and malaria, becoming increasingly resistant to medications. Lower-respiratory infections, diarrheal diseases, and measles appear to have peaked, at least temporarily.

Chen and Berlinguer argue that the traditional tripartite classification of disease—communicable diseases, noncommunicable diseases, and injury—appears to be breaking down. "New health threats are being superimposed on traditional diseases, driven at least in part by the forces of globalization. Globalization, thus, is generating epidemiological diversity and complexity" (Chen and Berlinguer 2001, 36).

Although mutating pathogens may account for some of the resurgence and spread of infectious disease, just as important have been the changes in social, political, and economic behaviors. Some two million people move across international borders each day. Some pathogens can reach anywhere in the world within 24 hours (Chen and Berlinguer 2001, 37). Whole populations are frequently displaced by civil war, ethnic conflict, or severe environmental degradation. Refugee camps are breeding grounds for disease. Urbanization can also stimulate the spread of disease: some cities lack the infrastructure to support rapid growth, and people often live close together without water or sewage treatment. Diseases can evolve in crowded prisons and then gain a foothold in communities. Patterns of individual behavior, such as unprotected sex and multiple partners, have been related to economic dislocation, driven in part by development. Environmental degradation (with resultant migration), combined with gender inequalities, has also been a key factor in the spread of disease, particularly HIV/AIDS (Lurie, Hintzen, and Lowe 1995; Kim, Millen, Irwin, and Gershman 2000). As noted in Chapter 2, climate change is thought to be a significant factor in the resurgence of infectious disease. Warmer temperatures and increased rainfall will probably increase and shift the geographic range of vectors such as mosquitoes.

Understanding, monitoring, and treating emerging infections will require global cooperation. So, too, will dealing with resistance to existing drug therapies. As public-health workers continue to address local health problems, they will need increasingly to think about their global aspects.

The spread of HIV and tuberculosis has called attention to the close relationship between microbiological disease and poverty (Farmer 1999). The prevalence of tuberculosis has long been a symptom of poverty, and the spread of HIV has been most rapid among impoverished and undernourished populations. Poverty not only damages the health of the poor, it makes the poor a health hazard to themselves and others by harboring and fostering mutations of infectious diseases (Grady 1996).

Poverty and Health

During the last century, human health has improved "more than during the entire previous span of human history" (World Bank 1994, 1). Average worldwide life expectancy increased from 48 years in 1955 to 66 years in 1998. During the same period, infant mortality declined from 155 to 59 per 1,000 live births, and about half as many children die before they reach the age of five. More people have adequate food, housing, sanitation, and education. Access to family planning has vastly improved. Specific health advances have included the elimination of smallpox and a reduction in the rate of polio infection.

But large disparities in health status also lurk, disparities both among and within nations. Sharp declines in life expectancy during the 1990s have been recorded, for example, in parts of sub-Saharan Africa and in the Russian Federation (Evans et al. 2001; Leon and Walt 2001). Infant mortality rates in the world's poorest countries are still 25 to 30 times higher than those of the wealthiest countries. Child mortality rates are about 40 to 60 times higher, and, most striking, maternal mortality is 750 to 1000 times higher than in countries with the lowest rates. Wide disparities within countries persist not only in the developing world but also in the most affluent nations such as the United States and Sweden. In the United States, for example, a comparison of counties with highest and lowest morality rates nationwide showed "a 13-year gap in women's life expectancy and a 16-year gap for men's" (Evans et al. 2001, 3) (see note 1).

In 1998, Gro Harlem Bruntland, the Director-General of the World Health Organization said,

Never have so many had such broad and advanced access to healthcare. But never have so many been denied access to health. The developing world carries 90 percent of the disease burden, yet poorer countries have access to only 10 percent of the resources that go to health.

(Quoted in Kim, Millen, Irwin, and Gershman 2000, 4)

It is apparent in this more troubling side of the health picture that, although many people have ridden high on a wave of economic growth, prosperity, and improved health, the rising tide has swept over vast expanses of humanity and sometimes caught them in the undertow. Poverty is perhaps the most important factor influencing health in the world today. Consider the results of the *Global Burden of Disease Study* (GBD). Begun in 1992 and finished four and a half years later, this study profiled the causes of death and morbidity around the world and attempted to make consistent comparisons among national regions (Murray and Lopez 1996). The GBD study reviewed over one-fourth of the death certificates in 1990 for the roughly 50.5 million individuals who died in that year. The diseases leading the list tended to be associated with regional poverty: lower-respiratory infections, diarrheal diseases, conditions arising during the perinatal period, and unipolar major depression, which is extremely widespread in the Southern hemisphere. The study also examined risk factors for disease and found that malnutrition led the list, with 11.7% of total deaths and 15.9% of DALYs. The next-most-important causes, also associated with regional poverty, were poor water supply, lack of sanitation, and unhygienic conditions. Unsafe sex followed, and was associated, along with other factors, with lack of education and lack of money for prophylaxis.

Ill health as a manifestation of poverty is to be found in a wide variety of forms. For example, the number of people homeless and moving within or across national borders continues to be extremely high. People on the move have few material goods and few resources for taking care of their health. They are also politically and materially dependent on the goodwill and services of others. They are often migrating as a result of changes in land ownership, as small peasant farmers are driven off land converted to production for market. Often coming from environments with which they and their cultures were well integrated, they seek refuge in new and unfriendly environments. They are forced to live in endless shanty towns, where millions of children sleep on the streets; they scavenge, beg, steal, and are victimized or murdered. In these crowded and unhygienic conditions, yaws, yellow fever, tuberculosis, malaria, and sexually transmitted diseases are on the rise. Poverty combined with inequality is everywhere contributing to the spread of infections (Farmer 1999).

There is increasing evidence that income distribution is an important determinant of health, and that health-care services are much more effective when they are distributed equally and within an egalitarian society (Braveman and Tarimo 2002; Marmot 2002; Kawachi and Kennedy 2002). Richard Wilkinson studied income equality and health empirically in First World countries (Wilkinson 1992; 1996): health status correlated weakly with wealth, but correlated strongly with economic equality. The more egalitarian the country, the healthier its population. There are many reasons for thinking this to be correct: inequality tends to increase poverty, which affects health more strongly than increasing wealth; diseases harbored in poverty tend to spread to all of society; inequalities create envy and stress harmful to health; health-care systems serving the whole population more or less equally provide appropriate services more widely and efficiently; and, according to some, wealth itself creates poverty by distorting the value of goods and sequestering basic resources for the wealthy (Gorz 1980).

Over the scale of income from absolute poverty to adequacy, income is by far the strongest predictor of health. Above a certain level of wealth, the relationship between wealth and health weakens: the curve, steep at the lowest levels of income, approaches horizontal at higher levels (World Bank 1993, 34). The shape of this curve tends to suggest that the notion of income *adequacy*, or meeting needs, is a sensible one. So, when considering the basic concept of justice, it is important to emphasize that with regard to public health, meeting the needs of the worst-off plays a key role in using resources efficiently to maximize the welfare of everyone (Elster 1992, 240; Rawls 1971, 60–61).

Poverty, Health, and Environment

Poverty is a basic determinant of health, and being sick or disabled increases the chance that poverty will take hold. Poverty and environmental decline are connected in a similar vicious circle—the more degraded an environment becomes, the fewer essential services it can provide, and the less it can support human health. The poor lack the luxury of moving to more hospitable places, nor can they buy clean water and safe food. Forced to live in degraded environments, their presence puts an additional strain on nature. As a result, the poor generally feel the worst effects of environmental degradation. If environmental decline continues apace, the world's poor will experience increasing trouble.

Consider, for example, food availability. Hunger and malnutrition are everywhere a serious problem. In the United States alone, some 11.2 million people cannot adequately feed themselves or their families, and in the developing world, 828 million people are chronically undernourished. About half of the 31,000 deaths of children under five every day are from hunger-related causes (Kim, Millen, Irwin, and Gershman 2000, 5). As we saw in Chapter 2, various environmental trends have the potential to further challenge food production around the world.

Although data on the international flow of toxic waste is imprecise, the pattern is clearly from North to South. Poor countries agree to import hazardous waste, often euphemistically labeled "recyclables," for money. These countries often have few health and environmental regulations, and the dangers of the materials being imported are not always well understood. Because facilities and standards are so primitive, workers often wear no protective gear such as gloves and masks, and they develop a number of health problems associated, for example, with exposure to lead, dioxin, mercury, and pesticides. Whole communities are put at risk because these "recycling facilities" often pollute the surrounding air, water, and soil. As regulations on hazardous waste in developed nations have grown increasingly strict over the past two decades, the flow of materials to the Third World has increased. The more regulations there are, the more expensive it is for a company to deal with waste, thus providing even more incentive to look for cheap foreign dumping grounds.

Economic Globalization and Health

Globalization is the rapid economic, political, and social integration that has occurred particularly in the past two decades. The free movement across national borders of capital, trade goods, people, ideas, and values has complex reverberations for health and environment. Some commentators whose work is focused on global health equity are highly critical of globalization (for example, Kim, Millen, Irwin, and Gershman 2000). They claim that it has significantly worsened the plight of the poor. Most are more cautious, often using such images as "the double face of globalization" (Yach and Bettcher 1998a). Evans et al., in their recent book on globalization and health conclude, "Whether its potential is effectively harnessed or its threats duly delivered remains to be seen" (Evans et al. 2001, 10).

There is concern among these authors that globalization is increasing poverty and worsening income disparities both within and among nations. Not only does the trend toward increased inequality and poverty portend declining public-health conditions, but the privatization of markets and capital has often resulted in fewer public funds for investment in health, education, and environmental protection. Some international corporations have begun to view the decline in availability and quality of key resources such as water as opportunities to make profits by controlling what was formerly in the commons.

According to an article by Gill Walt in *The Lancet*, the global liberalization of trade poses a number of health risks. Some of the potential risks include "the international trade in illegal products and contaminated foodstuffs, inconsistent safety standards, and the indiscriminate spread of medical technologies" (Walt 1998, 436). Unsafe products may make their way into all corners of the world. Consider tobacco. The lowering of trade barriers has allowed tobacco companies to export their products aggressively and to make use of global communication to advertise and market their products to previously untouched areas. The spread of tobacco globally has correlated, so far, with the spread of respiratory illness around the world. The Global Burden of Disease study projects that DALYs from tobacco use will skyrocket in the next decades, well above deaths from HIV or diarrhea (Murray and Lopez 1996, 742). Land that could otherwise be used to raise food is used instead to raise the tobacco crop, and wood is used to cure the leaf. Harmful chemicals such as methyl bromide and ethylene dibromide are used in processing (Yach 1996, 31). The moral involvement of the North in this particular plague may go beyond simply supporting and profiting from companies building these markets. An editorial in *The Lancet* noted that large providers of health insurance also maintain major investments in tobacco (Boyd, Himmelstein, and Woolhandler 1995).

Another effect of increased liberalization of trade has been a flow of low-wage industries to Southern-hemisphere countries. Labor standards in some regions are often deplorable—low wages, unsafe working conditions, and widespread child labor. The International Labor Organization estimated that in the mid-1990s the number of working children in the world increased from 80 million to 250 million (Bacon 1996, 30).

In the mid-1990s, a photographic exhibition of the work of Sebastião Salgado circulated in many cities (Salgado 1993). It depicted the working conditions of people around the world whose labor supplies the raw materials that make industrially based civilization possible. These photographs show that although hundreds of millions of people work in decent offices, factories, and homes, there are hundreds of millions in dangerous and dirty jobs paying subsistence wages. As industrialization expands, the number of these jobs is increasing. Working conditions that Americans like to think are the mark of nineteenth-century factories and sweatshops persist on a wider scale than ever before. Industries are moving to areas where costs are cheaper, in part because health and environmental regulations are less strict. The pressures for maximized productivity and profit lead to ecological decline, including the loss of genetic diversity and the spread of genetically modified organisms.

Philosophers generally hold the principle of justice to be most applicable under conditions of scarcity. As globalization increases economic inequality, it tends to aggravate the illusion among the world's consumer class that there is no scarcity, since they are themselves surrounded by goods and wealth imported from more deprived regions, of which they have learned to avoid notice (Mariner 1995). Even some of the most vocal proponents of fairness and equality in health care sometimes deny that scarcity is real: "The wealth of the world has not dried up; it has simply become unavailable to those who need it most" (Farmer 1999, xxvi). Perhaps *scarcity* is the wrong term, since it invites debate over when resources will finally completely "run out." Plenty of less-controversial vocabulary is available for describing the global environmental situation—such terms as *failing, insufficient,* and *in default* to future generations. These concepts embody the philosophical equivalent of scarcity.

Incongruous Health Services

As with other aspects of globalization, the globalization of the health-care service sector seems to have both positive and negative potential. Trends include the rise of medical tourism, migration of providers from lower-income to higher-income countries, foreign investment by pharmaceutical companies, the penetration of private markets into health services, the neglect of research and development regarding the so-called orphan diseases afflicting the poor, and iatrogenesis due to inappropriate application of new and often expensive health technologies (Evans et al. 2001). Increased privatization of health services has prompted a trend toward tertiary care, with reduced emphasis on preventive and primary care.

Problems arise from the general incongruity between Northern technology and Southern health needs. Southern elites often imitate Northern medical styles. Using the latest equipment, some cities build hospitals that emphasize treatment of the conditions of the wealthy. Local medical ethics discussions sound like those in the United States and Europe. As one prominent physician working in international primary care put it, medicine in poorer regions of the world strives to be a "photocopy" of First World medicine. Striving to lead and influence the world in its technological achievements, U.S. medicine fosters this mirroring.

Some high-tech procedures are appropriate for so few conditions that their global cost-effectiveness is questionable. Northern equipment often adapts poorly to the less developed world. So much infrastructure in the way of tools, power, and skills is needed to support Northern medical techniques that Southern efforts to copy technological medicine often fall far short of efficacy; old and broken equipment, inappropriate instructions, and sterile equipment in unsterile rooms too often characterize health services. This problem of incongruity is not confined to international comparisons. Because of the great contrast in wealth between the rich and the poor in the United States, complex technologies are often poorly suited to the neighborhoods they serve. Home dialysis, home tube feeding, and other such services place extreme burdens on households to provide appropriate electricity, sterilization, drainage, storage, time, and attention.

Private, for-profit, transnational hospital corporations also suffer from problems of incongruity. U.S. hospital chains are beginning to establish international networks. At the end of 1987 (the most recent figures we could find), there were 125 hospitals operated by corporations seated in other countries; 103 of these were U.S.-based, situated in 18 countries. The numbers have been increasing (Stocker, Waitzkin, and Iriart 1999; Jayachandran, Chandran, and O'Hara 1992, 184). Such institutions have some advantages: they build international commercial networks that can supplement United Nations and government enterprises, and they have strong commitments to economic efficiency. But since each region has different customs and needs, it is hard for centrally managed systems to provide locally responsive care. So far, such hospitals, by directing their services to middle-class and wealthy markets, have drawn private support away from public systems. As evidenced by their U.S. practices, these managed-care organizations lack commitment to equality and universal access (Jaychandran, Chandran, and O'Hara 1992, 187). Such systems may also offend local values; many cultures disdain health care for profit (Onoge 1975).

Pharmaceutical companies also may display some incongruity in their practices. There is concern over what appear to be a number of double standards for human subject research in the developing world. Beyond the issues of consent, questions have been raised about doing drug research on populations who probably will never be able to afford the drugs being tested on them. Pharmaceutical companies tend to ignore some of the major diseases of the developing world: although tropical diseases account for some 10% of the global disease burden, only 1% of the new drugs approved over the past quarter century have been for these diseases (Ford and Torreele 2001).

In the balance, bioethicists ought to oppose internationalization of U.S. health services until a thoroughgoing reexamination of our health-care technologies and organization has been undertaken. Consider the enthusias⸍ ⍳ of a study group at RAND, who proposed a new "Marshall Plan" for world health based on U.S. medical technology. They see an "unmatched opportunity" to "shape a world congenial to the United States" with health and health care as "a centerpiece of U.S. foreign policy" (Hunter, Anthony, and Lurie 2002). If such efforts are to succeed in improving global health, a much more modest model of U.S. health services needs to be worked out. The Green Health Center as described in Chapter 5, for example, would address both local and global health and justice concerns more effectively than current U.S. health services.

Moral Responses to the Global Situation

Good Health at Low Cost

We have argued throughout this book that the wealthier regions of the world need to live on an environmentally more modest budget that includes their health care. Can the world maintain good health while establishing environmentally less damaging and simpler ways of life? How might this be done? To answer this question, first keep in mind the relationship between population health and wealth: at high levels of income, health is relatively invariant with regard to wealth; at low levels of income, healthiness falls steeply with increasing poverty. It is thus important to prevent populations, or sectors of populations, from becoming so poor that the public-health infrastructure breaks down. This is one reason the concepts of sustainability and justice must be conceptually linked: modesty of consumption now can do much to protect future generations from unhealthy poverty.

In imagining a healthy, environmentally more modest society, it is important that it be a world in which environmental health underlies human health and where an integrated system of public-health measures is in place—not a world in which the health pyramid becomes very top-heavy, with environmentally expensive health-care measures for a few substituting for less costly and more widespread public health and environmental health.

Public-health measures need to be environmentally cost-effective. For example, in drier areas it may not make sense to maintain environmentally expensive water-based sanitation systems; latrine-composting systems for human waste might work better in the long run. Indeed, in planning for the worldwide hotter, drier environment that is entailed in climate change, perhaps these measures should be considered in long-range plans for some areas now served by water-based sewage systems. And as many have pointed out, a vegetarian diet is both healthier and environmentally less expensive than a diet heavy in meat.

In a more modest world, public-health fundamentals have high value. Because they are often built into other activities, many of them can be provided at little added cost as part of programs that pursue other social aims as well. For example, health education that would be costly to establish by itself fits well into a basic public literacy program. Safer transportation can be designed that is simultaneously less environmentally expensive than the American highway system.

Identifying the key elements of public health becomes more pressing as one considers scenarios of improved public health in regions of the world facing great scarcity ("We have no money, so we must think." [Maxwell 1985, 938]). A number of low-income countries have excellent public health status. In Sri Lanka, Costa Rica, China, Paraguay, Morrocco, and the Kerala State of India, where average income is a fraction of U.S. income, life expectancy at birth is higher than would be expected from income alone, and in some of these nations life expectancy is within a few years of U.S. levels (World Bank 1993, 54; Halstead, Walsh, and Warren 1985). Studies of these regions suggest synergistic effects of public health. They maintain much of the spectrum of public-health basics taken for granted in wealthier countries. Features include adequate nutrition, clothing, and shelter; essential health information; safe workplaces and public spaces; cleanliness and other restrictions on the spread of disease; sewage disposal and recycling; adequate quantities of water; low pollution levels; meaningful work; freedom from armed conflict; basic primary health care including vaccination programs and family planning; health-related research; professional education, surveillance, regulation, and record-keeping; a culture supportive of basic health rights; public involvement in health planning; and universal access to these services, resources, and activities (derived from Levy 1997).

What among these and other factors seems to stand out in the poor but healthy regions? John Caldwell and others identify a number of noteworthy factors (Caldwell 1986):

- *Women's autonomy, equality, and education.* Besides having a key role in their own health, women are usually important in perinatal health and the welfare of children. Women have traditions of attentiveness to health concerns. Protection of women's rights also increases the opportunity for women to work, to protect themselves in relationships, and to work in health-related services.
- *Substantial social commitment to education.* Good health requires education, and good health is needed for quality education. Commitment to women's education is important as a part of the commitment to education.
- *Universal access to primary health-care services.* Modest levels of medical intervention and relatively simple health-care technologies are significant in maintain-

ing good public health generally. Indeed, a less expensive system can more easily be made available to all. The density and efficiency of services is important, including household visits, perinatal care, and immunization campaigns.

- *Egalitarianism.* Populism creates pressure on governments and businesses to provide equal universal access to education and health services. This spirit also supports equality of women, and is consistent with justice as a key factor in sustainable health. Caldwell notes that populism and a radical spirit seem to be important health factors in both open and authoritarian societies by helping to extend the effects of health services to the whole population and reducing the proportion of the population that is poor and less able to benefit from health interventions. (Caldwell 1986, 200)

Where there is a commitment to public health as well as universal modest health care, the tolerance for expensive care for the rich is weakened. If one is unwilling to accept such a political outlook, then one has a responsibility to offer an alternative way to maintain a high level of public health and universal health care sustainably.

Access in a Global Context

Once one recognizes the global framework for making judgments regarding justice, the nationally limited perspective of the field of American bioethics falls into sharp relief. Although bioethicists have generally given strong and sometimes passionate support to universal access to health care, their attention to inequities has generally been confined to disparities within U.S. borders. This is understandable, since the focus of much bioethics discussion is on shaping national policy for the delivery of health services—a single political system is more manageable than the globe. Lack of insured access is so great in the United States that introduction of global concerns seems to introduce even more frustrating obstacles.

But more might be gained than is first evident by taking a global perspective, where a modest proposal such as the GHC could be seen as a model form of practice, not just as the lower tier of a multiclass system of access. Although Americans seem sleepily to accept extraordinary inequalities in income and wealth in most realms of life, they refuse to accept a double or multiple standard in access to health care as a moral norm. Our markedly unequal system of delivery derives not from a lack of a sense of justice, but from allowing responsiveness to individual and corporate autonomy to outweigh the concern for equality (World Health Organization 2000, 155).

A global perspective on justice supports a single standard of care. Instead of the poor receiving all forms of care the wealthy feel entitled to, a single standard requires that we move toward more modest services for the wealthy. The GHC is one step in that direction. It allows patients to choose to join the GHC voluntarily and caregivers to experiment with the practical problems of establishing limits.

There can be no justification in a sustainable world for an open-ended policy of providing environmentally costly services to patients simply because they can pay for them; the sorts of services offered by the GHC should become the standard for all classes of patients. This position contrasts with a common agenda in bioethics to argue for more services for the poor without challenging unlimited service to the wealthiest patients (Priester 1992, 93).

Reconciling Conflicts

Do principles of global justice and responsibility require that health systems be internationalized? Or that the U.S. medical system should perform extensive therapy and services abroad? No. The first responsibility of American health care is to the health of its own people. Fulfilling this role responsibly and with a strong sense of our global context provides the first and most significant step to fulfilling international responsibilities.

The aim should be neither to make the U.S. health care system like Southern systems nor to make Southern systems like the U.S. system. Just and sustainable care resembles neither. Fresh public and environmental health approaches are needed throughout the world. Insofar as American medicine revises its own practice in response to environmental and public health concerns, it will cut down on extreme procedures and revise technologies to make them more modest in resource consumption. Its medical model for the world can thereby become increasingly appropriate for a wide range of economic circumstances. Imitation, interconnection, and cooperation can then be more successful.

Consider the case of tuberculosis, one of the most widespread disease burdens in the world. Perhaps a third of the world's population carries TB, although many fewer are actively ill with it. Almost three million people die of TB and its attendant effects each year, and in the developing world most of these deaths occur in mid-life (Kochi 1991, 1–2). Drug-resistant TB infection, partly associated with the spread of HIV, is entering the germ pool. Epidemiologists believe that TB naturally tends to decline in a healthy human population (Enarson et al. 1995), as it did in Britain and Europe when nutrition improved during the last century or so (McKeown 1979). The advance of TB reflects spreading poverty and poor nutrition around the world.

Three strategies have been proposed for coping with TB: (*1*), a massive campaign of therapy; (*2*), selective therapy campaigns focused on health workers, HIV patients, and other selected populations; (*3*), general commitment to economic equality and adequate diets worldwide.

A universal program of therapy is problematic: present medications for TB are effective and not very expensive, but they require strict compliance from patients who must take pills daily or at longer intervals over months. Moreover, the growing immunity of TB to existing therapies is narrowing the temporal window for eradicating TB. In a world of declining health and shrinking resources, a massive therapy campaign is unlikely to succeed, and pharmaceutical companies are unlikely to commit resources to treat diseases whose primary sufferers are impoverished (Jameton 1995).

The second strategy, selective campaigns, is an obvious compromise—treatment of health workers, for example, is a key hindrance to the spread of the disease and, hopefully, development of therapies can ride the front of the wave of drug-resistant TB.

The third option, commitment to economic equality, admittedly overdetermines the result. It suggests Steve Martin's joke on a step-by-step approach to earning a million dollars: "First, get a million dollars." But it is the most likely to be successful in the long run and is justified by its many additional positive effects on health and morality. If it were not the case that modest consumption and greater equality are necessary to meet the environmental crisis, this would be an impractical alternative, but since redesign of wealth is a condition of coping with environmental change, we should recognize some of the health benefits that could be obtained through large economic and organizational changes.

Although the first responsibility of health professionals in the United States is to fulfill their global responsibilities by acting locally, international networks of care are valuable and could be strengthened. The World Health Organization is being underfunded by restructured world economies that hinder nations' ability to support the United Nations. Political ambivalence in the United States toward the U.N. and international service has hindered U.S. commitment to many of WHO's programs. WHO itself has in the past been dominated by First World physicians, when balanced worldwide representation could better serve planning.

Generally, Northern nations, and the United States in particular, need in their own regions to respect the ethical ground rules of the international organizations they are part of. It sometimes appears that international commitments to public health are merely for Southern consumption, and the Northern world is somehow exempt from its own good advice. It would have been interesting to see how much better the Alma-Ata Health For All campaign (WHO 1978) might have done if the commitment to primary care and universal access had been supported as the main approach to U.S. medical services.

Conclusion

Even if many international projects are limited in their effects, or are distorted by economic and political agendas other than health, these efforts are also educational for everyone involved. It is useful therefore for health professionals to spend time working in other countries in order to develop a better perspective on their own systems and to share both knowledge and ignorance. The bottom line is that if the United States were to make a local commitment to serve sustainable health, economic equality, and community participation, it would better serve global health as well.

Note for Chapter 7

1. Environmental Justice

Our topic here is an extension of the set of considerations forwarded more often under the heading of "environmental justice." *Environmental justice* usually refers to concern for the fair distribution of environmental burdens—sources of pollution, landfills, incinerators, toxic-waste dumps, smelters, refineries, or "locally undesirable land uses" (LULUs)—usually within U.S. borders (Bullard 1995, 6). Research done in the 1980s reveals that hazardous-waste facilities are disproportionately located in poor and minority neighborhoods. These inequalities affect the poor at several levels. Farm workers and their children may be exposed to toxic levels of pesticides in the fields, but they may also be exposed in their homes near the fields.

The related concept "environmental racism" makes the connection between environmentalism and civil rights explicit. A 1987 United Church of Christ study showed that race is the single most important predictor of the location of a hazardous-waste site. The study found that U.S. minorities were twice as likely as non-minorities to live near a hazardous facility, and three times as likely, as compared to non-minorities, to live near two or more such facilities (Westra and Wenz 1995, xv). A 1990 study by Argonne National Laboratory found that in the 136 U.S. counties where two or more air pollutants exceeded standards, resident populations were 33 percent white, 50 percent black, and 60 percent Hispanic (Bullard 1995, 4).

8

New Ways of Thinking About Bioethics

Since the field of bioethics emerged some four decades ago, much has changed in the world of health care and in the larger world that health care serves. The most important of these changes—the increasingly stressed state of the global ecosystem and the attendant decline in both ecosystem and human health—have immense relevance to health care. In its 40-year life, bioethics has proven itself a resilient and responsive field, able to stay abreast of the moral dimensions of technological and organizational changes within medicine. Mirroring the insularity of medicine, however, bioethics so far has not integrated environmental concerns into its dominant theoretical approaches. Nevertheless, we are hopeful that it will continue to transform its ways of thinking, and that it will become a vocal public advocate for the movement toward sustainable health by drawing forth the profound connections between health and the natural world.

Ethics seeks to answer the question "How ought we to live?" Throughout this book, we have been outlining the moral problems facing us at this period in human history, the values needed in response, and the moral stance that makes it possible to see some central problems clearly. An abundance of empirical information links health and environment. For the many people who strive to live a good life, a moral framework is needed to establish the relevance of this information, particularly for those thinking about the good life in the context of health care. Because the thinking that has thus far shaped bioethics has limitations that hold back this move toward sustainability, while environmental ethics has explored how to widen the circle of moral perception to include nature, a dialogue between the two is necessary and should prove fruitful.

What Might Environmental Philosophy Offer to Bioethics?

In 1967, historian Lynn White, Jr., published an article in *Science* entitled "The Historic Roots of Our Ecologic Crisis" (White 1967). White argued that one reason the environmental crisis has developed is that Christianity fostered a belief that nature exists solely as a resource for humans. Societies exploit nature partly because their religious and philosophical traditions regard the natural world as little more than a vast collection of raw materials. Since the 1960s, a rich and perceptive body of literature has developed around this question of how the dominant worldview, the conglomeration of beliefs and attitudes about nature that has developed within Western thought, shapes our troubled relationship to nature (Devall and Sessions 1985; Lopez 1990; Merchant 1985; Passmore 1974; Thomas 1996).

Like many other contemporary scholars, William Leiss argues that destructive attitudes toward nature were crystallized during the Enlightenment by the development of modern science, which gave birth to the dream that humans would achieve complete mastery over nature. Philosophy rationalized and legitimized the drive to master nature: the sharp division of the world into spiritual (the human mind, the noumenal world) and material (nature, the phenomenal world) encouraged humans to view nature as usable machinery, without any spiritual animation. The growth of capitalism, particularly the agenda of increasing human material well-being by exploiting natural resources, was closely tied to this philosophical trend (Leiss 1994, xx).

According to Leiss, mastery over nature "has been a more or less tacit presupposition of modern ideologies within their systems of explicit rationalization for concepts such as individual freedom, social justice, economic development through market forces, imperialism, and élite or class privilege" (Leiss 1994, xx). Humanity's entitlement to dominate nature, "a subterranean theme that runs throughout the collective consciousness of the modern era" (Leiss 1994, xviii), is a grounding presupposition of the moral philosophy that has shaped bioethics. Although scholars in bioethics have challenged a number of tacit assumptions in modern philosophy's theoretical edifice, the exploitative attitude toward nature has seldom been one of them.

As the field of environmental ethics developed during the 1970s and 1980s, and as environmental problems became more pronounced, environmental philosophers began to challenge these assumptions about the human relationship to nature and to see that the concepts and methods of philosophy were themselves limiting factors in adequately addressing environmental problems. Philosophers began to explore more radical approaches: *biocentrism*, for example, which argues that all

living things deserve moral consideration; and *ecocentrism*, which moves attention to the value of whole ecosystems. A more comprehensive overview of environmental philosophy as it relates to bioethics also includes *deep ecology*, *social
ecology*, and *ecofeminism*.

Biocentrism

Paul Taylor characterizes biocentrism as "biocentric egalitarianism": in principle,
all living beings have equal inherent worth and an equal right to pursue their own
form of flourishing. A life-centered ethic, in contrast to an anthropocentric one,
entails "prima facie moral obligations that are owed to wild plants and animals
themselves as members of Earth's biotic community" (Taylor 1981, 160). Other
things being equal, humans are morally bound to protect wild plants and animals
or promote their good for their own sake. Our duties to protect biodiversity, to
seek to maintain balance in ecosystems, and to slow global warming are rooted in
obligations to individual entities.

The ground of the obligation to protect and promote the good of living entities
stems, in Taylor's theory, from two interconnected concepts that together are the
basis of respect for nature. First, every organism has a good of its own, which
humans—the only moral agents—can either thwart or promote by our actions.
This good Taylor defines as the full development of an entity's "biological
powers," or its capacity to cope with its environment and live out its full life
cycle (161). Compare this rich notion of an entity's good to the standard debate
about animal research, which connects the good of a living thing almost entirely
to its sentience or its capacity to feel pain.

The second of Taylor's key concepts is that of inherent worth. A living entity
is worthy of being preserved for its own sake and therefore deserves moral consideration. Taylor draws a parallel between an attitude in human ethics of respect
for persons and in environmental ethics of respect for nature. "When we adopt an
attitude of respect for persons as the proper (fitting, appropriate) attitude to take
toward all persons as persons, we consider the fulfillment of the basic interests of
each individual to have intrinsic value" (162). The attitude of respect for nature is
an ultimate or fundamental commitment—there is no higher norm to which it
refers. As Taylor says, "It sets the total framework for our responsibilities toward
the natural world" (161).

When Taylor says that in principle all living things have equal inherent worth,
the "in principle" clause is an admission that we will act out of preference for our
own species and that this is morally acceptable. Taylor deals with this pervasive
paradox by suggesting that obligations to other living things

are entirely additional to and independent of the obligations we owe to our fellow humans.
Although many of the actions that fulfill one set of obligations will also fulfill the other,
two different grounds of obligation are involved. . . . If we were to accept a life-centered

theory of environmental ethics, a profound reordering of our moral universe would take place. . . . Our duties with respect to the "world" of nature would be seen as making prima facie claims upon us to be balanced against our duties with respect to the "world" of civilization (160).

Ecocentrism

Ecocentrism, or *holism*, is the view that the biosphere as an interconnected whole has moral standing. Beginning from the science of ecology, it sees the world as an integrated web of parts and relationships. One cannot sensibly value just "life" or the lives of individual creatures only, as in biocentrism, because the whole organic process involves death and decay. There must be some other locus of value. Homeostasis, equilibrium, and integrity are normative principles from which we can derive our obligations to nature. In Aldo Leopold's now famous phrase, "A thing is right when it tends to preserve the integrity, stability, and beauty of the biotic community. It is wrong when it tends otherwise" (Leopold 1949, 224–225).

The roots of Leopold's "land ethic," which he articulated in the final chapter of *A Sand County Almanac*, lie in evolutionary theory and ecology. Influenced by David Hume and Adam Smith, Charles Darwin argued that ethics rests upon human "sentiments." The bonds of familial and parental affections are shared by all mammals, and this expanded circle of social sentiments proved to be an effective adaptive strategy for the human species. "All ethics so far evolved," says Leopold, "rest upon a single premise: that the individual is a member of a community of interdependent parts" (203). As we come to understand (through ecology) our connection to the biotic community, it is natural that our moral sentiments should extend to it. "The land ethic simply enlarges the boundaries of the community to include soils, waters, plants, and animals, or collectively: the land . . ." (204)

Leopold grounds his land ethic in what he calls "ecological conscience." We can be ethical, he says, only in relation to "something we can see, feel, understand, love, or otherwise have faith in" (214). Leopold uses the story of Odysseus to argue this point: When Odysseus returned from Troy, he hanged a dozen female slaves whom he suspected of betraying him. For Odysseus, this was an ethical course of action, since slaves were property, not people. Similarly, many today fail to extend moral obligation to the land because they see it as mere property. Just as our moral sensibilities have expanded to include all humans, we need to extend the moral community to include the land upon which and within which we live. So the first task in talking about responsibilities to nature is to establish nature as something we can see, feel, understand, and love.

Ecocentrism does not displace responsibilities to individual entities, including people, but incorporates them—though holistic concerns may take priority. Leopold and other ecocentrists have used a metaphor of tree rings, or expanding concentric circles, and argued for the accretion of new, larger rings, with duties to human community, especially to family, forming the core.

Naturalistic Ethics

Many philosophers, and others, distrust biocentrism, ecocentrism, and other naturalistic approaches to ethics; "Nature" is a hook on which deep fears about humans' place in the world seem to snag. The most serious worry seems to be that to give nature moral worth is somehow to devalue humans.

Stephen J. Gould argues that scientific revolution occurs in two stages: a realignment of concepts of the physical universe (the easy part) and a reassessment of human status (the hard part). As if the shift from a geocentric to a heliocentric universe, and the loss of our cosmic standing, were not enough, Darwinism "robbed man of his particular privilege of having been specially created, and relegated him to descent from the animal world" (Gould 1998, 68, quoting Sigmund Freud). Although informed people almost universally accept the physical construction of the living world implied by the theory of evolution, they dispute its implications for humanity.

The main thrust of environmental philosophy is the completion of this revolution. Fears that some important notion of dignity or "soul" may be threatened are certainly legitimate. "Naturalistic" ethics can and has been put to ill use: the concept of "nature" has played some vicious ideological roles in relation to gender, sexual orientation, and race. But there is no necessary progression from Darwinism to a devaluing of humans. Insofar as evolutionary theory is, given what we know now, a scientifically accurate picture of ourselves, it must be consistent with a relatively accurate picture of human obligations.

The wealth of ecologically related principles presented in this and previous chapters (especially Chapter 5) promises great potential for extending the agenda of bioethics. The ecological perspective on ethics allows the ethics of health care to cohere with a more relevant ethic guiding human conduct generally during this century of globalization and environmental crisis, and helps avoid a concentration on the conduct of health professionals and patients isolated from the larger changes in our global condition. Grounding human morality in an ecological framework radically alters our relationships to each other and to the larger biotic community. It leads us to identify different, often new, moral problems and facilitates the movement toward a culture that respects nature's limits, that consumes modestly and shares nature's now-fragile bounty broadly, deeply, and convivially. It is within this kind of worldview that the notion of sustainable health will most comfortably find a home. But this wealth of new ideas challenges the essential drive in philosophical theory for parsimony of concepts and principles in philosophical theory.

Unity and Plurality in Ethics

Stephen Toulmin has argued that medicine saved the life of ethics (Toulmin 1982). At a time when the academic discipline was stagnating, philosophers, theologians, and other academicians found purpose in helping health professionals cope with the rapid and morally complex changes in their world. Practical challenges forced the revitalization of theoretical work. New thinking, both applied and theoretical, expanded to embrace not only medicine but also business, environment, journalism, politics, education, and a host of other professions. Yet this diversity of ethics, given the prevailing modern notion that all values are relative to the individual, has also had the unfortunate effect of fragmenting theory and diminishing our sense of commonality and theoretical unity. Bioethics, along with the other academic splinters of ethics, needs to seek a more unified ecological moral framework that bases analysis and application on its ability to "preserve the ecosystems which sustain it" (Elliott 1997).

The first major enterprise in medical ethics, and perhaps the project that most helped it coalesce into a coherent discipline, resulted from an act of Congress establishing the National Commission for the Protection of Human Subjects of Biomedical and Behavioral Research. Its best-known publication, *The Belmont Report*, published in 1979, set forth three principles to guide the ethical conduct of research: respect for persons, beneficence, and justice. As Albert Jonsen remembers it, these three principles "came to mind almost unbidden" (Baker et al. 1999, 266). Because the principles were fluid and offered a framework for exploring moral problems rather than a rigid moral calculus, they served well the discussion of dilemmas created by rapid technological change in medicine. Medical ethics had discovered itself.

Although these concepts are vague (Takala 2001), retaining this common vocabulary serves a practical purpose as bioethics takes on the more inclusive moral challenges of our deteriorating habitat. Problem-solving application of accepted principles and methods to new situations and conditions can begin immediately. Without much reflection on theory or principles, bioethicists, clinicians, and patients can more intuitively integrate a fresh consciousness of their global situation that might lead them to make different decisions simply because their understanding of the facts is so different. For example, patients might be more willing to limit care; clinicians might gently discourage expensive care that simply prolongs dying; ethicists might write more about problems relating to materials and services. The principles and grounding of ethics will not have changed dramatically, only our perception of the reality around us.

The central principles that have thus far guided bioethics remain relevant, though specification of the principles will need to reflect awareness of environmental responsibility. Beauchamp and Childress argue that "specification holds out the possibility of a continually expanding normative viewpoint that is faithful to ini-

tial beliefs (which are not renounced) and that tightens rather than weakens coherence among the full range of accepted norms." (Beauchamp and Childress 1994,
31) Norms are not, as they note, meant to be static, but can evolve and find shape
as we face new moral dilemmas, or as our perceptions of old moral dilemmas
change. The norms widely accepted in medical ethics discussion and practice can
evolve in response to the environmental challenge.

Just as a core set of values evolved to respond to the needs of the developing
field of bioethics, another set has evolved in environmental ethics. This book represents our effort to press for the integration of key environmental value into the
discussion of bioethics: sustainability, a fair distribution of environmental benefits and burdens, modesty of consumption, responsibility to nature and to future
generations. In our view, this set of principles, the principles of sustainability,
should become central guiding principles of discussion in health-care ethics. So,
we propose here to discuss how the conventional framework might effectively be
modified by and integrated with ecological concepts.

Beneficence and Nonmaleficence

Health Care Without Harm, which campaigns to reduce toxic hospital wastes, uses
as its slogan "First, do no harm." Although HCWH's practical agenda is conservative—for example, better separation of health-care wastes, phase-out of health-
care products containing polyvinyl chloride (PVC)—their use of the principle of
nonmaleficence is actually quite radical, and takes the principle far beyond its
traditional functions in medical ethics. "Do no harm," suggests that health professionals' responsibilities to avoid harm extend beyond the bedside and beyond
the health-care setting. Health professionals must avoid harming the community
and the natural environment.

Likewise, the principle of beneficence, which has been used in bioethics to
inform doing good for the patient, takes on a much different meaning when used
in an environmental context. If a clinician must take into account not only his or
her patient's good, but also the good of the factory worker who assembled the
thermometer that the nurse is reading, and the good of those who might be exposed to the waste products of the thermometer once it is discarded, the range of
application of the principle has broadened dramatically.

Bioethics has certainly explored issues where beneficence and nonmaleficence
extend beyond the bedside. The sticky problem of quarantine for individuals with
infectious illness such as tuberculosis raises the issue of preventing harm to the
community. Childhood vaccinations usually pose small risks to a child in exchange
for protecting the community's health as well as the child's. Some bioethicists
have raised the question of whether physicians have obligations to the community at large, with actions such as working to prevent human rights abuses or providing free or low-cost care for the poor.

Bioethics has not yet seriously grappled with the background volume of harm, both practical and philosophical, brought to attention by the environmental discussion. Although there is discussion in the biomedical literature about how best to define harm, there is a broad level of implicit agreement that, in the context of medicine, *harms* can only be done to humans. The same assumption underlies the principle of doing good. These presuppositions lay out a moral system in which nonhuman forms of life, as well as inanimate nature, lack moral value. They may be relevant to a discussion about morality, but only in their utility or disutility to humans. Animal research is the only bioethics context we are aware of in which nonmaleficence has been extended beyond our own species.

Strong responsibilities to the environment *can* be established within a strictly "human-centered" view. Global warming, for example, poses potential risks of grave harm to humans, regardless of whether we care about the survival of nature *per se* (although of course we are dependent on it as well). But there are compelling reasons for considering a more robust understanding of harms and benefits.

The public, together with most of us in bioethics, usually celebrates the technological benefits and promise of medicine as though they were separable from the destructiveness of the society that supports health care and helped compensate for it. But Western civilization, especially in the United States, is probably the most destructive civilization in the history of humankind. This destructiveness cannot be appreciated fully if we focus largely on the short-term interests of individuals and their immediate communities, as we normally do when we consider beneficence and nonmaleficence in bioethics. According to environmental ethics, additional considerations must be taken into account: the good of future human generations, of people around the world, of nonhuman species, and of earth's ecosystems, which are collective entities that cannot be reduced to the individuals that compose them.

Moreover, the harm that we are doing is mostly a collective harm. If we examine each individual decision one by one, we usually highlight the benefits to be achieved in the care of a single patient, and we discount or disregard the harm done during the life cycle of the materials we use to achieve this good. In so doing, we are acting like sensible utilitarians and choosing an action where the good clearly seems to outweigh the costs. But in doing so, we are also adopting, as ethicists, a consumerist perspective that gives moral weight only to one link of the whole chain of consequences of an action. Since health care, and society at large, collectively causes harm of a similar kind millions of times over, (such as carbon emissions and toxic waste) each tiny bit of harm adds up to the great cumulative disaster of climate change and the global ecological crisis.

When we realize that the technology of health care—which can be neither developed nor applied without intensive use of oil, mining, and chemistry, with all their side effects—is environmentally destructive, we must recognize that our normal way of assessing beneficence disregards the precariousness of the earth's situation and its relationship to the technology of medicine. Worse, we are unable to do so in part because of our anthropocentrism.

When the full cost to the life of the earth is put into the balance, everyday decisions unquestioned by ethicists and regarded as rational and even praiseworthy may be seen as questionable and possibly maleficent. If nonmaleficence is viewed from an environmental perspective in the form of the precautionary principle, many health care activities probably do at least as much harm to the world as good (Kohn, Corrigan, and Donaldson 2000).

Autonomy, Coercion, and Participation

Autonomy has not always held the primacy of place in philosophy that it now commands in bioethics. In early moral philosophy, personal autonomy was not central but functioned, in Albert Jonsen's words, as a "prop for arguments about moral accountability and responsibility" since there had to be some sense of free will in order to make humans responsible for their own actions (in Baker et al. 1999, 268). Even Kant, who is often hailed as the father of autonomy, bound it to a concept of universal law determining human decisions. Yet autonomy has gradually taken hold as the moral trump card in much contemporary work in bioethics. The principle of autonomy, in its modern form, articulates the core commitment of liberal theory to personal freedom and to the idea that individuals have the right to make choices for themselves, based on their own values and goals. Now environmental questions challenge both the standard meaning of autonomy and its primacy of place in bioethics.

There are several respects in which environmental concerns press for a more nuanced principle of autonomy. The tension that was implicit in the notion of autonomy as understood by Kant and others needs to be rediscovered. Autonomous individuals exist as members of a moral community who share common ends. This community needs to expand to place humans within their biotic community. With a shift in thinking, personal choice can be understood in the context of belonging to and feeling responsible to the biological as well as the human community.

Some may suspect that this reframing of autonomy is an attempt to sugar-coat certain forms of coercion. Perhaps, within health care, there is some truth to this. A sustainable health-care system will undoubtedly limit the choices of both patients and physicians. But patients and physicians alike are already coerced by prevailing interventionist standards and by the ready availability of heroic "life-saving" treatments and drugs. And people already need to be coaxed and prodded into healthier lifestyles, conserving health-care products, and forgoing expensive and marginally useful treatments. It may turn out that there is no increase in the level of coercion, if its direction shifts from forcing expansion to supporting stewardship and modest health-care consumption.

For the concept of autonomy to be richly nuanced so that it can guide respect for human dignity while avoiding its crude application as a catch-all for personal choice, it must be placed in proper relationship to the concept of connection. *Connection*, or interdependency, is a common motif in the environmental literature. The images of circularity, balance, and webs recur frequently, both as description and as normative ideals. Ecology is based on the study of connections between elements in a living system, including humans. Todd and Todd speak of human enterprises being "coevolutionary with the natural world" (Todd and Todd, xiv). The world is a "whole Earth community." Principles of ecological design prioritize "working with nature" and "harmony with nature": connection is built into design, with closed loops of production, waste transformed into energy, and humans integrated into biotic communities.

Although in conventional bioethics obligations derive from the sincere convictions of the autonomous individual, the ecological concept of obligation is more intimately grounded in connection than is autonomy. Connectedness is about "binding" and is closely related to the idea of community; communities are a stronger ground of obligation than the beliefs of individuals. Inclusion in a community is the main source of moral obligation (see Leopold 1949). Not only does the idea of interconnection place us in community, but it also expands the concept of community. From an ecological perspective, we are global citizens and members of a biotic community.

If one's "self" is defined by and through relationships, this connectedness can also be seen as being at odds with conceptions of the self as autonomous. Both feminist and environmental writings have explored such interconnected conceptions of the self (see, e.g., Benhabib 1992; Naess 1989). Environmental philosophers amplify this alternative view by suggesting that the "self" is more appropriately defined through relationship not only with other people, but also with nature. Warwick Fox's *Toward a Transpersonal Ecology* is the most sustained treatment of the "ecological self." One of the more interesting implications of a "transpersonal self" (a "wide, expansive, or field-like conception of the self") is that: "Care flows naturally if the 'self' is widened and deepened so that protection of free Nature is felt and conceived as protection of ourselves. . . ." (Fox quoting Arne Naess 1990, 217)

It is tempting to romanticize the idea of humans in community with nature, but nature plays a significant role in unpleasant human experiences of disease, suffering, and death. Humans are hosts to a vast number of parasites living in our intestines, on our skin, in our hair. Many of these interrelationships are symbiotic and quite necessary to our health, while others we rightly label as diseases. Yet even disease, as biologist René Dubos is famous for saying, is part of the overall harmony of nature. It is important that while treating the disease element as an intruder, we think ecologically: the most obvious tie that binds us with the rest of life is the inevitability of death, disease, and decay. It has already been well argued in bioethics that we need not equate death with failure and that palliation of suffering should sometimes outweigh efforts to save lives. An ecological perspective adds to this argument the ability to make death more meaningful in a large biological context.

Nevertheless, the expression of self-control—of controlling desires for material goods, of making choices in light of the needs of the whole community—is a clear and strong expression of self-determination. So how should the individual be included in an ecological perspective on health-care decision-making? A shift in thinking needs to occur so that the articulation of personal choice is understood inside the context of duties to each other and to nature. Autonomy is not necessarily threatened by this contextualization: individual choice can be an expression of belonging in and feeling responsible to the human and biological community.

For autonomy to be maximized in a sustainable context, individuals need to be able to participate, and feel that they are participating, in the decisions that set social priorities to protect humans and nature. The language of individual participation is similar to the language of individual autonomy. Both concepts offer the patient a voice in health-care decisions. But the language of participation is more communitarian; it lacks the implications of individual separateness found in the language of autonomy. Where clinician and consumer disagree, for example, the language of autonomy leads to a power struggle over whose opinion should dominate. Indeed, "Who should decide?" has been one of the major questions in health-care ethics. In contrast, the language of participation is a language of inclusion. The question of who should decide, then, can be answered flexibly, depending on what needs to be decided.

Justice, Equality, and Balance

Basic political and material equality is a prominent feature of the modern concept of justice. Yet, for several reasons, an ecological point of view does not so obviously entail equality (Dobson 1998). Even though all people face a common global environmental dilemma, people in different regions and conditions experience this circumstance very differently. Nor is saying that we are all interconnected to say that we are all equal. If strict material equality were insisted upon, and the ability of the environment to support human life fell to a low level, then survival and equality would become mutually inconsistent. Even in good times, the ideal of equality fits poorly with basic concepts of ecological community. Since animals and plants are part of our community, we need to consider the fundamental differences among species as basic to rules on how to treat them. Given the distinctness of the ecological roles of species and their radically differing capacities for pleasure and pain, it is probably best not to use equality as the central concept for understanding justice in the whole ecological community.

In the world of nature, however, the concept of justice has a close affinity to the Platonic ideal of justice as harmony. A healthy ecosystem is one that *justifies*—that is, balances or harmonizes—the complex relationships among its components. Since all creatures in an ecosystem are interdependent, attributing excessively high standing to a conscious élite of large organisms is problematic unless the élite, like Plato's guardians, are living modestly and thinking of the welfare of the whole.

These classical conceptions of justice also connect human health to justice. A healthy person's body is also a "just" one, with its harmony and temperance realized as homeostasis. In this sense ecological medicine contains a commitment to justice, and bioethics can reframe the problem of justice as an effort to balance the fundamental elements of ecological balance: preservation of ecosystems, maintenance of community and population health, and care for the individual. A healthy and sustainable balance of resources allocated among these three spheres would be a just one as well.

Philosophers writing about justice in health care have often focused on distinctions that acquiesce in dissimilar treatment of individuals. Once that step has been taken, there is little in doctrines of equality to make it clear that extreme differences in allocation of resources are problematic. But if we accept the principle that everyone in the world has an equal claim to the earth's commons and resources, then we can justly claim that everyone has an equal entitlement to the use of Earth's atmosphere, so the agenda of equalizing industrial output of carbon becomes one of central moral significance. The concept of justice as balance then comes into play. Rather than leaving ourselves without a way of attacking extreme disparities that stem from the principle of autonomy, we can hold that for the sake of harmony and balance, only small differences in access to resources should be tolerated.

Are sustainability and justice necessarily related? If one omits concern for the welfare and interests of future generations, then one can imagine an unsustainable world that meets the criteria of justice for a short time. This world may be efficient, meet people's needs, and allocate resources and power equally, but only until Earth's ecosystem collapses. If one believes that justice includes the needs and interests of future generations, however, then a just world must also be sustainable. To state the relationship the other way around, if the world is unsustainable then it is also unfair, at least to future generations and to nature's great ecosystem.

There are additional connections and disconnections between sustainability and justice. The most obvious is efficiency in the use of global resources. Since the largest sustainable gains in efficiency can be achieved by leveling down consumption by those who are well off, and the pressure for reducing overall consumption is great, greater material equality is the surest route to sustainability (Daily and Ehrlich 1995). This strategy is consistent with a Rawlsian perspective on justice.

Rawls argued that it was morally acceptable to allocate more resources to some people if it in fact helped the condition of the worst off (Rawls 1971). He made this argument with the assumption that economic growth would result; but in the contracting economy, growth is economically impossible, and thus Rawls must be run in reverse: we must first take from the better off in order to increase resources available to the worst off.

The potential conflict between meeting basic human needs and preserving nature presents a difficult practical challenge for environmentalism. Holmes Rolston III raises poignant questions about meeting the needs of the poor when doing so may involve wiping out habitat for tigers (Rolston 1996). But if the needs of the poor are to be met for any extended period of time, it is necessary to preserve the ecological stability of the regions where they live. A right to environmental protection should be regarded as one element of basic human rights, since a sound ecology is also a condition of human health (Sachs 1995; 1996). As with the Rawlsian argument, this means that economic change during the environmental crisis must involve a combination of leveling down of wealth and income for the best off with a leveling up of the worst off.

Justice and Modesty

Bioethics has dwelt primarily on the medical problems of individuals in clinical settings—more specifically, on the moral questions that arise in academic medical centers. The clinical setting has controlled the discourse. As we note above, this narrowly focused gaze limits opportunities to discuss crucial questions about the environment and about justice, questions that are inherent in contemporary medical procedures and technologies. Ethical conversation about justice in the access of patients to therapies has tended to focus on the benefits and monetary costs to individuals and their families; more distant environmental expenditures in the life cycle of medical products recede to the background.

The parameters of bioethical discussion of high-cost therapies were set about 40 years ago in the Seattle debate over access to dialysis. Machines were too scarce and their use too expensive for distribution to all who needed them. The question of justice centered on *deservingness*. Bioethicists criticized allocation criteria explicitly based on merit, behavior, or social class, and on the whole supported criteria such as medical need or prospects for recovery. But these more neutral principles still resulted in a vast disparity in the levels of health care available to different economic classes. The exclusion of some people from services, and the inclusion of others, remains a premise underlying the discussion of justice in medical care.

Working for the most part in medical centers with highly paid health professionals, and addressing the clinical problems of patients able to afford them, bioethicists have tended to accept wide differences in care and have been willing to perform philosophical work that justifies those differences. A more global perspective opens the prospect of grappling with what Paul Farmer labels "the leading ethical question of our times"—the immense disparities in public health around the world (Farmer 2003, 204).

But environmental philosophies are ready at hand to save the moral life of bioethics. Such philosophies generally view overconsumption as not only destructive of our habitat but a moral failing in itself, and they prescribe *modesty* as a tonic for the spiritual emptiness engendered by the endless pursuit of material goods. The permaculture ethic, for example, calls for "active conservation, ethics and frugal use of resources, and 'right livelihood.'" Deep ecology promotes a philosophy of "simple in means, rich in ends." The writings of Thoreau are an early articulation of voluntary simplicity. A surprisingly widespread desire to live modestly is evidenced by the popularity of Duane Elgin's book *Voluntary Simplicity*, first published in 1981 (Elgin). It advocates three interconnected tenets: frugal consumption, ecological awareness, and personal growth. Like permaculture and deep ecology, voluntary simplicity responds to the need to protect nature and at the same time heals the malaise of a materialistic lifestyle. By consuming less and worrying less about what we want to buy, we have more time and energy to spend with our children, family, and friends and to enjoy games, music, and other wholesome activities. It is only a small step to conclude that a simple life requires a modest system of medical care.

The notion of *modesty* is about having "enough." But what is enough? The question suggests why the element of personal growth is considered a central tenet of simple living. Maturity is marked by the ability to distinguish between needs and desires, and between personal and community needs.

Conclusion

A viable bioethics informed by environmental philosophy will

- be able to include an account of the value of the natural world,
- have some mechanism for balancing human health needs with the needs of nature,
- appreciate that the proper context of bioethics is global in scope,
- commit us to a strong principle of justice that demands a leveling in the distribution of resources and risks, and that aims toward modesty and adequacy for all, and
- have ecological sustainability as a core evaluative principle.

Those who are attuned to the state of our planetary health and to the living conditions of people around the world may feel an overwhelming sense of helplessness and hopelessness. The problems humanity faces seem so complex and so serious that it is hard know how—or even whether—to take action. Our inevitable complicity in the death of nature and the suffering of distant others may cause so much moral discomfort that simple avoidance seems the only psychologically bearable response.

But it is not necessary to adopt a stance of despair. Millions of people around the world are working toward reconciling human needs with the limits of the earth. All of us have a moral responsibility to become aware of how our actions affect others globally, human and nonhuman alike, and how our daily lives are likely to shape the future. We have a responsibility to educate ourselves and others, and to do some careful thinking about what we need and do not need, who we care about, and how we mean to care for them. If we feel a commitment to promoting and maintaining human health, we must take the state of the natural environment immediately and carefully into account. We must embrace sustainable health for humans and for the ecosystems we depend on for survival.

Bibliography

1992. *United Nations Conference on Environment and Development; 1992 June 1–12; Rio de Janeiro*. Washington, D.C.: Council on Environmental Quality.

1994. Population: The View from Cairo. *Science* 265:1164–7.

Abramovitz, Janet N. 2001. Averting Unnatural Disasters. In *State of the World 2001*, edited by L. R. Brown, C. Flavin and H. French. New York: W. W. Norton & Company.

Academy of Medical-Surgical Nurses. 2002. *AMSN Official Position Statement on: Code of Conduct/Ethics* 2002 [accessed December 29, 2002]. Available from www.med surgnurse.org/default.htm.

Achtenberg, Ben (Producer); and Ann Carol Grossman (Director). 1995. *No Time to Waste*. Boston: Fanlight Productions. Videotape (29 minutes).

Agency for Toxic Substances & Disease Registry. 1997. ToxFAQs for Mercury.

Aiken, William; and LaFollette, Hugh. 1996. *World Hunger and Morality*, Second ed. Upper Saddle River, New Jersey: Prentice Hall.

Allaby, Michael. 2000. *The Environment: An Inside Look*. Milwaukee, Wisconsin: Gareth Stevens.

American Academy of Dermatology. 2001. *Ethics in Medical Practice, Principles of Professional Conduct* [accessed January 2, 2003]. Available from www.aadassociation.org/ethics.html.

American Association of Respiratory Care. 2002. *Statement of Ethics and Professional Conduct* 1994 [accessed December 29 2002]. Available from www.aarc.org/media_center/position_statements/ethics.html.

American Council on Science and Health. 1999. *Review and Consensus Statement—A Scientific Evaluation of Health Effects of Two Plasticizers Used in Medical Devices and Toys: A Report from the American Council on Science and Health*. Medscape General Medicine [accessed June 22, 1999]. http://www.medscape.com/.

127

American Holistic Nurses' Association. 2002. *Code of Ethics for Holistic Nurses* 2002 [accessed December 29, 2002]. Available from www.ahna.org/about/statements.htm l#ethics.

American Medical Association. 2002. *Principles of Medical Ethics, June 2001* [accessed December 29, 2002]. Available from www.ama-assn.org/ama/pub/category/2512.html.

American Public Health Association. 2002. *2002* [accessed December 29, 2002]. Available from www.apha.org.

Ames, Steven. 1994. *A Guide to Community Visioning: Hands-on Information for Local Communities*. Third ed. Portland: Oregon Visions Project of the American Planning Association's Oregon Chapter.

Anand, Sudhir; and Amartya K. Sen. 1996. *Sustainable Human Development: Concepts and Priorities*. New York: United Nations Development Programme.

Annas, George. 1995. Reframing the Debate on Health Care Reform by Replacing Our Metaphors. *New England Journal of Medicine* 332(11):745–8.

Anastas, Paul T.; and J. C. Warner. 1998. *Green Chemistry, Theory and Practice*. New York: Oxford University Press.

Argyle, Michael. 1987. *The Psychology of Happiness*. London: Methuen & Co. Ltd.

Ashford, Lori; Interim Working Group on Reproductive Health Community Security; and United States Agency for International Development. 2002. *Securing Future Supplies for Family Planning and HIV/AIDS Prevention* [accessed January 4, 2003]. www.prb.org.

Athanasiou, Tom. 1996. *Divided Planet: The Ecology of Rich and Poor*. Boston: Little, Brown and Company.

Attfield, Robin. 1983. *The Ethics of Environmental Concern*. New York: Columbia University Press.

———. 1999. *The Ethics of the Global Environment*. West Lafayette, Indiana: Purdue University Press.

Bacon, David. 1997. Still Hungry: A Report on the World Food Summit in Rome, Italy. *Z Magazine* 10(1):28–31.

Baker, J. T.; R. P. Borris; B. Carte; G. A. Cordell; and D. D. Soejarto, et al. 1995. Natural Product Drug Discovery and Development—New Perspectives on International Collaboration. *Journal of Natural Products* 58(9):1325–57.

Baker, Robert. 1998. A Theory of International Bioethics: Multiculturalism, Postmodernism, and the Backruptcy of Fundamentalism. *Kennedy Institute of Ethics Journal* 8(3): 201–31.

———. 1999. Negotiating International Bioethics: A Response to Tom Beauchamp and Ruth Macklin. *Kennedy Institute of Ethics Journal* 8(4):423–53.

Baker, Robert B.; Arthur L. Caplan; Linda L. Emanuel; and Stephen R. Latham, eds. 1999. *The American Medical Ethics Revolution: How the AMA's Code of Ethics Has Transformed Physicians' Relationships to Patients, Professionals, and Society*. Baltimore: The Johns Hopkins University Press.

Beauchamp, Tom L. 1999. A Mettle of Moral Fundamentalism. *Kennedy Institute of Ethics Journal* 8(4):389–401.

Beauchamp, Tom L.; and James F. Childress. 1994. *Principles of Biomedical Ethics*. Fourth ed. New York: Oxford University Press.

———. 2001. *Principles of Biomedical Ethics*. Fifth ed. New York: Oxford University Press.

Beck, Ulrich. 1999. *World Risk Society*. Cambridge, Massachusetts: Polity Press.

Bell, Simon; and Stephen Morse. 1999. *Sustainability Indicators: Measuring the Immeasurable*. London: Earthscan Publishers.

Benhabib, Seyla. 1992. *Situating the Self: Gender, Community, and Postmodernism in Contemporary Ethics*. New York: Routledge.

Benyus, Janine M. 1997. *Biomimicry: Innovation Inspired by Nature*. New York: William Morrow and Co., Inc.

Berlinguer, G. 1999. Globalization and Global Health. *International Journal of Health Services* 29(3):579–95.

Berrill, Norman. 1955. *Man's Emerging Mind*. New York: Dodd, Mead and Co.

Birch, Charles; and John B. Cobb, Jr. 1981. *The Liberation of Life: From the Cell to the Community*. Cambridge: Cambridge University Press.

Bocock, Robert. 1993. *Consumption*. New York: Routledge.

Bodenheimer, T. 1997a. The Oregon Health Plan—Lessons for the Nation (first of two parts). *New England Journal of Medicine* 337(9):651–5.

———. 1997b. The Oregon Health Plan—Lessons for the Nation (second of two parts). *New England Journal of Medicine* 337(10):720–3.

Bongaarts, John. 1996. Population Pressure and the Food Supply System in the Developing World. *Population and Development Review* 22(3):483–503.

Booth, Ken; Tim Dunne; and Michael Cox, eds. 2001. *How Might We Live? Global Ethics in the New Century*. Cambridge: Cambridge University Press.

Borrini, Grazia. 1992. Environment and "Health as a Sustainable State": Concepts, Terms and Resources for a Primary Health Care Manager in Developing Countries. Rome: International Course for Primary Health Care Managers at District Level in Developing Countries, Instituto Superiore di Sanita.

Borrini-Feyerabend, Grazia. 1995. Promoting Health as a Sustainable State. *Medicine and Global Survival*:162–75.

Bouvier, Leon F.; and Jane T. Bertrand. 1999. *World Population: Challenges for the 21st Century*. Santa Ana, California: Seven Locks Press.

Boyd, Wesley J.; David U. Himmelstein; and Steffie Woolhandler. 1995. Commentary: The Tobacco–Health Insurance Connection. *Lancet* 346(8976):64.

Boyden, Stephen; and Stephen Dovers. 1992. Natural-Resource Consumption and Its Environmental Impacts in the Western World. Impacts of Increasing Per Capita Consumption. *Ambio* 21(1):63–9.

Boylan, Michael, ed. 2001. *Environmental Ethics*. Upper Saddle River, New Jersey: Prentice Hall.

Boyle, Alan E.; and Michael R. Anderson, eds. 1996. *Human Rights Approaches to Environmental Protection*. Oxford: Clarendon Press.

Branch, Michael; and Jessica Pierce. 1996. "Another Name for Health:" Thoreau and Modern Medicine. *Literature and Medicine* 15(1):129–45.

Braveman, Paula; and Eleuther Tarimo. 2002. Social Inequalities in Health Within Countries: Not Only an Issue for Affluent Nations. *Social Science and Medicine* 54:1621–35.

Brooks, David. 2000. The Way We Spend Now. *The New York Times Magazine*, 15 October 2000, sec. 6, col. 1, p. 55.

Brooks, Stuart M.; Michael Gochfeld; Jessica Herzstein; Richard J. Jackson; and Marc B. Schenker, eds. 1995. *Environmental Medicine*. St. Louis: Mosby.

Brown, Lester R. 1995. *Who Will Feed China? Wake Up Call for a Small Planet*. The Worldwatch Environmental Alert Series. New York: W. W. Norton & Company.

———. 2001. *Eco-Economy: Building an Economy for the Earth*. New York: W. W. Norton & Company.

———. 2001. Eradicating Hunger: A Growing Challenge. In *State of the World 2001*, edited by L. R. Brown, C. Flavin, H. French and others. New York: W. W. Norton & Company.

Brown, Lester R.; Christopher Flavin; and Hilary French, et al. 2001. *State of the World 2001*. New York: W.W. Norton & Company.

Brown, Lester R.; Gary Gardner; and Brian Halweil. 1998. *Beyond Malthus: Sixteen Dimensions of the Population Problem*. Edited by Linda Starke. Worldwatch Paper, 143. Washington, D.C.: Worldwatch Institute.

Bryant, Bunyan. 1995. *Environmental Justice: Issues, Policies, and Solutions*. Washington, D.C.: Island Press.

Buell, Lawrence. 2001. *Writing for an Endangered World: Literature, Culture, and Environment in the U.S. and Beyond*. Cambridge: Harvard University Press.

Bullard, Robert. 1990. *Dumping in Dixie: Race, Class, and Environmental Quality*. San Francisco: Westview.

———. 1995. Decision Making. In *Faces of Environmental Racism: Confronting Issues of Global Justice*, edited by Laura Westra and Peter S. Wenz. Lanham, Maryland: Rowman & Littlefield Publishers, Inc.

Bunch, Bryan. 1999. Chloracne. In *The Family Encyclopedia of Disease: A Complete and Concise Guide to Illnesses and Symptoms*. New York: Scientific Publishing Inc., W. H. Freeman and Company.

Bunyanavich, Supinda; and Ruth Walkup. 2001. U.S. Public Health Leaders Shift Toward a New Paradigm of Global Health. *American Journal of Public Health* 91(10): 1556–8.

Burger, Joanna. 1997. *Oil Spills*. New Brunswick, New Jersey: Rutgers University Press.

Butler, Colin D. 1991. Global Warming, Ecological Disruption, and Human Health. *Medical Journal of Australia* 155:351.

———. 1994. Overpopulation, Overconsumption, and Economics. *Lancet* 343:582–4.

Butman, C. A.; J. T. Carlton; and S. R. Palumbi. 1995. Whaling Effects on Deep-Sea Biodiversity. *Conservation Biology* 9:462–4.

Cairns, John Jr. 1997. Defining Goals and Conditions for a Sustainable World. *Environmental Health Perspectives* 105(11):1164–70.

———. 1999. The Quest for Increased Longevity on an Unsustainable Planet. *Ecosystem Health* 5(2):67–9.

Caldwell, John C. 1986. Routes to Low Mortality in Poor Countries. *Population and Development Review* 12(2):171–220.

Callahan, Daniel. 1990. *What Kind of Life: The Limits of Medical Progress*. New York: Simon and Schuster.

———. 1996. Can Nature Serve as a Moral Guide? *Hastings Center Report* 26(6):21–2.

———. 1998. *False Hopes: Why America's Quest for Perfect Health Is a Recipe for Failure*. New York: Simon & Schuster.

Caldicott, Helen. 1992. The Earth Is Dying: The Medical Implications of the Ecological Crisis. *Family Practice* 9(4):391–6.

Callicott, J. Baird. 1994. Toward a Global Environmental Ethic. In *Ethics and Agenda 21: Moral Implications of a Global Consensus*, edited by N. J. Brown and P. Quiblier. New York: United Nations Environment Programme, United Nations Publications.

———. 2002. An Ecocentric Environmental Ethic. In *Applying Ethics*, edited by John Olen and Vincent Barry. Belmont, California: Wadsworth.

Canadian Association of Physicians for the Environment. 2003. *Greening Health Care*. [accessed January 3, 2003]. Available from www.cape.ca/greening.html.

Capra, Fritjof. 1982. *The Turning Point: Science, Society, and the Rising Culture*. New York: Simon and Schuster.

———. 1996. *The Web of Life: A New Scientific Understanding of Living Systems*. New York: Anchor Books.

Carrick, Paul. 1999. Environmental Ethics and Medical Ethics: Some Implications for End-of-Life Care, Part I. *Cambridge Quarterly of Healthcare Ethics* 8(1):107–18.

Carson, Rachel. 1987, c1962. *Silent Spring.* Boston: Houghton Mifflin.

Catton, Jr., William R. 1982. *Overshoot: The Ecological Basis of Revolutionary Change.* Urbana: University of Illinois Press.

Chambers, Nicky; Craig Simmons; and Mathis Wackernagel. 2000. *Sharing Nature's Interest: Ecological Footprints as an Indicator of Sustainability.* London: Earthscan.

Chen, Lincoln C.; and Giovannit Belinguer. 2001. Health Equity in a Globalizing World. In *Challenging Inequities in Health: From Ethics to Action,* edited by T. Evans, M. Whitehead, F. Didderichsen, A. Bhuiya, and M. Wirth. New York: Oxford University Press.

Chesworth, Jennifer, ed. 1996. *The Ecology of Health.* Thousand Oaks, California: Sage Publications.

Chivian, Eric. 2001. Environment and Health: 7. Species Loss and Ecosystem Disruption—The Implications for Human Health. *Canadian Medical Association Journal* 164(1):66–9.

Chivian, Eric; Michael McCally; Howard Hu; and Andrew Haines. 1993. *Critical Condition: Human Health and the Environment.* Cambridge: MIT Press.

Clapp, Richard. 2000. Environment and Health: 4. Cancer. *Canadian Medical Association Journal* 163(8):1009–12.

Coates, Peter. 1998. *Nature: Western Attitudes Since Ancient Times.* Berkeley: University of California Press.

Cohen, Joel E. 1995a. *How Many People Can the Earth Support?* New York: W. W. Norton & Company.

———. 1995b. Population Growth and Earth's Human Carrying Capacity. *Science* 269:341–6.

Colborn, Theo; Dianne Dumanoski; and John P. Myers. 1996. *Our Stolen Future: Are We Threatening Our Fertility, Intelligence, and Survival—a Scientific Detective Story.* New York: Dutton.

Colborn, Theo; Frederick S. vom Saal; and Ana M. Soto. 1993. Developmental Effects of Endocrine-Disrupting Chemicals in Wildlife and Humans. *Environmental Health Perspectives* 101(5):378–84.

Collingwood, R. G. 1949. *The Idea of Nature.* Oxford: Clarendon Press.

Committee on Health Effects of Waste Incineration, Board on Environmental Studies and Toxicology, Commission on Life Sciences, and National Research Council. 2000. *Waste Incineration and Public Health.* Washington, D.C.: National Academy Press.

Costanza, Robert; Ralph d'Arge; Rudolf de Groot; Stephen Farber; Monica Grasso; Bruce Hannon; Karin Limburg; Shahid Naeem; Robert V. O'Neill; Jose Paruelo; Robert G. Raskin; Paul Sutton; and Marjan van den Belt. 1997. The Value of the World's Ecosystem Services and Natural Capital. *Nature* 387:253–57.

Cothern, C. Richard, ed. 1995. *Handbook for Environmental Risk Decision Making: Values, Perceptions, and Ethics.* Boca Raton, Florida: Lewis Publishers.

Crews, Frederick. 2001. Saving Us from Darwin. *New York Review of Books* XLVIII (15):24–31.

Daily, Gretchen, ed. 1997. *Nature's Services: Societal Dependence on Natural Ecosystems.* Washington, D.C.: Island Press.

Daily, Gretchen C.; and Katherine Ellison. 2002. *The New Economy of Nature.* Washington, D.C.: Island Press.

Daly, Herman. 1996. *Beyond Growth: The Economics of Sustainable Development.* Boston: Beacon Press.

Daniels, Norman. 1986. Why Saying No to patients in the United States Is So Hard: Cost Containment, Justice, and Provider Autonomy. *New England Journal of Medicine* 341(21):1380–3.

Danis, Marion; and Larry R. Churchill. 1991. Autonomy and the Common Weal. *Hastings Center Report.* 21(1):25–31.

Davies, Terry; and Adam I. Lowe. 1999. *Environmental Implications of the Health Care Sector.* Washington, D.C.: Resources for the Future.

de Gruijl, Frank R.; and Jan C. van der Leun. 2000. Environment and Health: 3. Ozone Depletion and Ultraviolet Radiation. *Canadian Medical Association Journal* 163(7):851–5.

De Villiers, Marq. 2000. *Water: The Fate of Our Most Precious Resource.* Boston: Houghton Mifflin Company.

de Waal, Frans. 1996. *Good Natured: The Origins of Right and Wrong in Humans and Other Animals.* Cambridge: Harvard University Press.

de-Shalit, Avner. 2000. *The Environment: Between Theory and Practice.* Oxford: Oxford University Press.

Denning, Jeannie. Phone interview with the Regulatory Affairs Manager at Hudson Respiratory Care Incorporated (RCI), Omaha, Nebraska. March 7, 2001.

Devall, Bill. 1988. *Simple in Means, Rich in Ends: Practicing Deep Ecology.* Lanyon, Utah: Gibbs Smith Publication.

Devall, Bill; and George Sessions. 1985. *Deep Ecology: Living As If Nature Mattered.* Lanyon, Utah: Gibbs Smith Publication.

Dobson, Andrew. 1998. *Justice and the Environment: Conceptions of Environmental Sustainability and Dimensions of Social Justice.* Oxford: Oxford University Press.

Dobson, Andrew, ed. 1999. *Fairness and Futurity: Essays on Environmental Sustainability and Justice.* New York: Oxford University Press.

Drummond, Ian; and Terry Marsden. 1999. *The Condition of Sustainability.* New York: Routledge.

Dubos, René. 1965. *Man Adapting.* New Haven: Yale University Press.

———. 1966. *Man and His Environment: Biomedical Knowledge and Social Action, Scientific Publication 131.* Washington, D.C.: Pan American Health Organization, World Health Organization.

———. 1968. *So Human an Animal.* New York: Charles Scribner's Sons.

Dubos, René; and Jean-Paul Encande. 1980. *Quest: Reflections on Medicine, Science, and Humanity.* Translated by Patricia Ranum. New York: Harcourt Brace Jovanovich.

Durning, Alan Thein. 1991. Asking How Much Is Enough. In *State of the World 1991: A Worldwatch Institute Report on Progress toward a Sustainable Society,* edited by Lester R. Brown. New York: W. W. Norton & Company.

———. 1992. *How Much Is Enough? The Consumer Society and the Future of the Earth.* New York: W. W. Norton & Company.

Eckholm, Erik. 2001. Then Came the Locusts: A Chinese Region Reels. *New York Times,* September 25, A4.

Ehrlich, Paul R.; Gretchen C. Daily; Norman Myers; and James Salzman. 1997. No Middle Way on the Environment. *The Atlantic Monthly,* 98–104.

Ekins, Paul. 1991. The Sustainable Consumer Society: A Contradiction in Terms? *International Environmental Affairs.* 3(4):243–58.

Eldredge, Niles. 1998. *Life in the Balance: Humanity and the Biodiversity Crisis.* Princeton: Princeton University Press.

Elgin, Duane. 1981. *Voluntary Simplicity: Toward a Way of Life That Is Outwardly Simple, Inwardly Rich.* New York: Morrow.

Elliott, Herschel. 2002. *A General Statement of the Tragedy of the Commons* 1997 [accessed November 6 2002]. Available from www.dieoff.com/page121.htm.

Elster, Jon. 1992. *Local Justice: How Institutions Allocate Scarce Goods and Necessary Burdens.* New York: Russell Sage Foundation.

Emanuel, Ezekial J. 1991. *The Ends of Human Life: Medical Ethics in a Liberal Polity.* Cambridge: Harvard University Press.

Enarson, D. A.; J. Grosset; E. Mwinga; S. Herschfield; R. O'Brian; S. Cole; and L. Reichman. 1995. The Challenge of Tuberculosis: Statements on Global Control and Prevention. *Lancet* 346:809–19.

Environmental Protection Agency. 1999. *Fact Sheet: Polychlorinated Dibenzo-p-dioxins and Related Compounds Update: Impact on Fish Advisories.* EPA-823-F-99-015; September.

———. 2000a. Exposure and Human Health Reassessment of 2,3,7,8–Tetrachlorodibenzo-p-Dioxin (TCDD) and Related Compounds. Washington, D.C.: Environmental Protection Agency.

———. 2000b. Questions and Answers about Dioxins: U.S. Environmental Protection Agency Office of Research and Development's Center for Environmental Assessment.

———. 2001. Dioxin: Database of Sources: U.S. Environmental Protection Agency Office of Research and Development's National Center for Environmental Assessment.

———. 2002. *Global Warming Site 2002* [accessed September 10, 2002]. Available from www.epa.gov/globalwarming/index.html.

Epstein, Helen. 2001. Time of Indifference. *New York Review of Books* 48 (6):33–42.

Evans, Robert G.; Morris L. Barer; and Theodore R. Marmor, eds. 1994. *Why Are Some People Healthy and Others Are Not? The Determinants of Health of Populations.* New York: Aldine de Gruyter.

Evans, Timothy; Margaret Whitehead; Finn Diderichsen; Abbas Bhuiya; and Meg Wirth, eds. 2001. *Challenging Inequities in Health: From Ethics to Action.* New York: Oxford University Press.

Evernden, Neil. 1992. *The Social Creation of Nature.* Baltimore: Johns Hopkins University Press.

Factor 10 Club. 2002. *Carnoules Declaration: 1994 Declaration of the Factor 10 Club* 1994 [accessed June 25, 2002]. Available from www.factorten.co.uk.

Farmer, Paul. 1999. *Infections and Inequalities: The Modern Plagues.* Updated edition. Berkeley: University of California Press.

———. 2001. The Major Infectious Diseases in the World—To Treat or Not to Treat. *New England Journal of Medicine* 345(3):208–10.

———. 2003. *Pathologies of Power.* Berkeley: University of California Press.

Flegal, Katherine M.; Margaret D. Carroll; Cynthia L. Ogden; and Clifford L. Johnson. 2002. Prevalence and Trends in Obesity among U.S. Adults, 1999–2000. *Journal of the American Medical Association* 288(14):1723–7.

Florida State University. 2002. *Taxol Research at FSU* [accessed November 24, 2002]. www.research.fsu.edu/taxol/discovery.html.

Foege, W. H. 1998. Global Public Health: Targeting Inequities. *Journal of the American Medical Association* 279(24):1931–2.

Ford, N.; and E. Torreele. 2001. Neglected Diseases of Global Importance. *Journal of the American Medical Association* 286(23):2943–4.

Fox, Daniel M.; and Jordan S. Kassalow. 2001. Making Health a Priority of U.S. Foreign Policy. *American Journal of Public Health* 91(10):1554–6.

Fox, J. E.; M. Starcevic; K. Y. Kow; M. E. Burow; and J. A. McLachland. 2001. Nitrogen Fixation: Endocrine Disruptors and Flavonoid Signalling. *Nature* 413:128–9.

Fox, Warwick. 1990. *Toward a Transpersonal Ecology: Developing New Foundations for Environmentalism*. Boston: Shambhala.

Freeman, Edward R.; Jessica Pierce; and Richard H. Dodd. 2000. *Environmentalism and the New Logic of Business*. New York: Oxford University Press.

Friedman, Emily. 1996. *The Right Thing: Ten Years of Ethics Columns from* The Healthcare Forum Journal. San Francisco: Jossey-Bass Publishers.

Frumkim, Howard. 2001. Beyond Toxicity: Human Health and the Natural Environment. *American Journal of Preventive Medicine* 20(3):234–40.

Garrett, Laurie. 1994. *The Coming Plague: Newly Emerging Diseases in a World Out of Balance*. New York: Farrar, Straus and Giroux.

Georgescu-Roegen, Nicholas. 1995. Summary of: The Entropy Law and the Economic Problem. In *A Survey of Ecological Economics*, edited by R. Krishnan, J. M. Harris, and N. R. Goodwin. Washington, D.C.: Island Press.

Germain, S. 2001–2002. The Ecological Footprint of Lions Gate Hospital. *Hospital Quarterly* 5(2):61–6.

Gillespie, Michael. 2002. Saving What We Love at Any Cost: The Rhetoric of Heroic Medicine as Diversion. *Journal of Medical Humanities* 23(1):73–86.

Girod, Jennifer. 2002. A Sustainable Medicine: Lessons from the Old Order Amish. *Journal of Medical Humanities* 23(1):31–42.

Glacken, Clarence J. 1967. *Traces on the Rhodian Shore: Nature and Culture in Western Thought from Ancient Times to the End of the Eighteenth Century*. Berkeley: University of California Press.

Glaspey, Jacob; Natalie Johnson; and Rachel Jameton. 2003. *Progress of Green Chemistry in Pharmaceutical Industry*. Unpublished manuscipt.

Golley, Frank B. 1998. *A Primer for Environmental Literacy*. New Haven: Yale University Press.

Goodland, Robert. 1992. The Case That the World Has Reached Limits. In *Population, Technology, and Lifestyle*, edited by R. Goodland, H. E. Daly, and S. El Sarafy. Washington, D.C.: Island Press.

Goodman, David C.; Elliot S. Fisher; George A. Little; Therese A. Stukel; Chiang-hua Chang; and Kenneth S. Schoendorf. 2002. The Relation Between the Availability of Neonatal Intensive Care and Neonatal Mortality. *New England Journal of Medicine* 346(20):1538–44.

Gorz, André. 1980. *The Poverty of Affluence*. Boston: South End Press.

Gould, Stephen J. 1998. Can We Complete Darwin's Revolution? In *The Environmental Ethics and Policy Book*, edited by D. VanDeVeer and C. Pierce. Belmont, California: Wadsworth.

Grady, Denise. 1996. Quick-Change Pathogens Gain an Evolutionary Edge. *Science* 274:1081.

Gray, Bradford H. 1992. World Blindness and the Medical Profession: Conflicting Medical Cultures and the Ethical Dilemmas of Helping. *The Milbank Quarterly*. 70:535–57.

Greenberg, Michael R., ed. 1987. *Public Health and the Environment*. New York: The Guilford Press.

Griffin, Donald R. 2001. *Animal Minds: Beyond Cognition to Consciousness*. Chicago: University of Chicago Press.

Grumbach, Kevin. 2002. Specialists, Technology, and Newborns—Too Much of a Good Thing. *New England Journal of Medicine* 346(20):1574–5.

Guillette, Louis J., Jr.; and Mark P. Gunderson. 2001. Alterations in Development of Reproductive and Endocrine Systems of Wildlife Populations Exposed to Endocrine-Disrupting Contaminants. *Reproduction.* 122:857–64.

Gunderson, Lance H.; C. S. Holling; and Stephen S. Light, eds. 1995. *Barriers and Bridges to the Renewal of Ecosystems and Institutions.* New York: Columbia University Press.

Haines, Andrew; Anthony J. McMichael; and Paul Epstein. 2000. Environment and Health: 2. Global Climate Change and Health. *Canadian Medical Association Journal* 163(6):729–34.

Halstead, Scott B.; Julia A. Walsh; and Kenneth S. Warren, eds. 1985. *Good Health at Low Cost.* New York: The Rockefeller Foundation.

Hanson, Mark; and Daniel Callahan. 1999. *The Goals of Medicine: The Forgotten Issues in Health Care Reform.* Washington, D.C.: Georgetown University Press.

Harvie, James. 1999. Eliminating Mercury Use in Hospital Laboratories: A Step Toward Zero Discharge. *Public Health Reports* 114.

Hawken, Paul; Amory Lovins; and L. Hunter Lovins. 1999. *Natural Capitalism: Creating the Next Industrial Revolution.* Boston: Little, Brown and Company.

Health Care Without Harm. 2000. *Heed the Warnings: Health Care Without Harm Calls for Action on PVC and DEHP in Medical Products* [accessed May 22, 2000]. Available from www.noharm.org.

———. 2002. *Aggregate Exposure to Phthalates in Humans* Health Care Without Harm, 2002 [accessed September 14, 2002]. Available from www.noharm.org.

Henderson, Hazel. 1996. *Building a Win-Win World: Life Beyond Global Economic Welfare.* San Francisco: Berrett-Koehler Publishers.

Heredia, Rudolf C. 1994. The Ethical Implications of Global Climate Change: A Third World Perspective. In *The Ethical Dimensions of the United Nations Program on Environment and Development, Agenda 21,* edited by Donald A. Brown, Conference Director. New York: United Nations.

Hertsgaard, Mark. 1999. *Earth Odyssey: Around the World in Search of our Environmental Future.* New York: Broadway Books.

Hille, John. 1998. *The Concept of Environmental Space: Implications for Policies, Environmental Reporting and Assessments.* Luxembourg: European Environment Agency.

Homer-Dixon, Thomas. 2000. *The Ingenuity Gap: How Can We Solve the Problems of the Future?* New York: Alfred A. Knopf.

Hunter, Robert E.; Anthony C. Ross; and Nicole Lurie. 2002. *Make World Health the New Marshall Plan* [accessed October 10, 2002]. www.rand.org.htm.

Ichiyo, Muto. 1998. Ecological Perspectives on Alternative Development: The Rainbow Plan. *CNS.* 9(1):3–23.

Institute for Food and Development Policy. 2001. Water as Commodity: The Wrong Prescription. *Food First Backgrounder* 7(3).

Institute of Medicine. 1997. *America's Vital Interest in Global Health.* Washington: National Academy Press.

Intergovernmental Panel on Climate Change. 2001a. *Climate Change 2001: Impacts, Adaptation, and Vulnerability. A Report of Working Group II of the Intergovernmental Panel on Climate Change.*

———. 2001b. *Summary for Policy Makers: A Report of Working Group I of the Intergovernmental Panel on Climate Change.*

International Association of Biomedical Laboratory Science. 2002. *Environmental Policy Statement 1998* [accessed December 29, 2002]. Available from www.iamlt.org/environment-pp.htm.

International Council of Nurses. 2002. *ICN Code of Ethics for Nurses 2000* [accessed December 29, 2002]. Available from www.icn.ch/ethics.htm.

International Federation of Red Cross and Red Crescent Societies. 2001. *World Disasters Report 2001* [accessed October 31, 2001]. Available from www.ifrc.org/publicat/wdr2001/intro.asp.

Jameton, Andrew. 2002. Outcome of the Ethical Implications of Earth's Limits for Health Care. *Journal of Medical Humanities* 23(1):43–60.

Jameton, Andrew; Catherine McGuire; and The Working Groups of the Green Health Center and Exploring Bioethics Upstream Project. 2002. Toward Sustainable Healthcare Services: Principles, Challenges, and a Process. *International Journal of Sustainability in Higher Education* 3(2):113–27.

Jameton, Andrew; and Jessica Pierce. 1997. Toward a Sustainable U.S. Health Policy: Local Congruities and Global Incongruities. *Social Indicators Research* 40:125–46.

Jameton, Rachel. 1995. IL-12 Possibilities. *Science* 269: 1498.

Jayachandran, C. R.; R. Chandran; and Lisa O'Hara. 1992. Internationalization of Multi Hospital Systems. *Journal of Hospital Marketing* 7(2):183–96.

Jenkins, Joseph. 1999. *The Humanure Handbook*. Second ed. Grove City, Pennsylvania: Jenkins Publishing.

Johnson, Lawrence E. 1991. *A Morally Deep World: An Essay on Moral Significance and Environmental Ethics*. Cambridge: Cambridge University Press.

Jonsen, Albert R.; Mark Siegler; and William J. Winslade. 1998. *Clinical Ethics: A Practical Approach to Ethical Decisions in Clincial Medicine*. Fourth ed. New York: McGraw-Hill, Health Professions Division.

Kass, Leon. 1983. The Case for Mortality. *The American Scholar*. 52(2):173–91.

Kauppi, Pekka. 1995. The United Nations Climate Convention: Unattainable or Irrelevant. *Science* 270(5241):1454.

Kawachi, Ichiro; and Bruce P. Kennedy. 2002. *The Health of Nations: Why Inequality Is Harmful to Your Health*. New York: The New Press.

Kennedy, Paul. 1993. *Preparing for the Twenty-First Century*. New York: Random House.

Khan, Kausar S. 1994. Epidemiology and Ethics: the Perspective of the Third World. *Journal of Public Health Policy*. 15(1):218–25.

Kilner, John F. 1990. *Who Lives? Who Dies? Ethical Criteria in Patient Selection*. New Haven: Yale University Press.

Kim, Jim Yong; Joyce V. Millen; Alec Irwin; and John Gershman, eds. 2000. *Dying for Growth: Global Inequality and the Health of the Poor*. Monroe, Maine: Common Courage Press.

King, Maurice. 1990a. Health Is a Sustainable State. *Lancet* 336(8716):664–7.

———. 1990b. Swellengrebel Lecture: Public Health and the Ethics of Sustainability. *Tropical and Geographical Medicine* 42:197–206.

King, Maurice; and Charles Elliott. 1993. Legitimate Double-Think. *Lancet* 341(8846): 669–72.

Klare, Michael. 2001. The New Geography of Conflict. *Foreign Affairs* 80(3):49–61.

Kochi, Arata. 1991. The Global Tuberculosis Situation and the New Control Strategy of the World Health Organization. *Tubercle* 72:1–6.

Kohn, Linda; Janet Corrigan; and Molla Donaldson, eds. 2000. *To Err Is Human: Building a Safer Health System*. Washington, D.C.: National Academy Press.

Kolata, Gina. 2002. Research Suggests More Health Care May Not Be Better. *The New York Times*, July 21, 1.

Kolpin, Dana W.; Edward T. Furlong; Michael T. Meyer; E. Michael Thurman; Steven D. Zaugg; Larry B. Barber; and Herbert T. Buxton. 2002. Pharmaceuticals, Hormones, and Other Organic Wastewater Contaminants in U.S. Streams, 1999–2000: A National Reconnaissance. *Environmental Science & Technology* 36(6): 1202–11.

Koop, C. Everett; Clarence E. Pearson; and Roy M. Schwarz, eds. 2001. *Critical Issues in Global Health*. San Francisco: Jossey-Bass.

Kroll-Smith, Steve; Phil Brown; and Valerie Gunter, eds. 2000. *Illness and the Environment: A Reader in Contested Medicine*. New York: New York University Press.

Kroll-Smith, Steve; and H. Hugh Floyd. 1997. *Bodies in Protest: Environmental Illness and the Struggle over Medical Knowledge*. New York: New York University Press.

Kübler-Ross, Elizabeth. 1969. *On Death and Dying*. New York: Macmillan.

Langhorne, Richard. 2001. *The Coming of Globalization*. New York: Palgrave.

Last, John. 1998. *Public Health and Human Ecology*. Second ed. Stamford, Connecticut: Appleton & Lange.

Lavastida, Jose I. 2000. *Health Care and the Common Good*. Lanham, Maryland: University Press of America.

Leaning, Jennifer. 2000. Environment and Health: 5. Impact of War. *Canadian Medical Association Journal* 163(9):1157–61.

Lee, Kai N. 1993. *Compass and Gyroscope: Integrating Science and Politics for the Environment*. Washington, D.C.: Island Press.

Leiss, William. 1994. *The Domination of Nature*. Montreal: McGill-Queen's University Press.

Leon, David A.; and Gill Walt, eds. 2001. *Poverty, Inequality, and Health: An International Perspective*. New York: Oxford University Press.

Leopold, Aldo. 1949. *A Sand County Almanac and Sketches Here and There*. New York: Oxford University Press.

Levit, Katharine; Cynthia Smith; Cathy Cowan; Helen Lazenby; and Anne Martin. 2002. Inflation Spurs Health Spending in 2000. *Health Affairs* 21(1):172–81.

Levy, Barry S. 1997. Conditions in Which People Can Be Healthy. *The Nation's Health* (*American Public Health Association*) 27(4):2.

Logie, Dorothy. 1992. The Great Exterminator of Children. *British Medical Journal*. May 30; 304:1423–6.

Lomborg, Bjørn. 1998. *The Skeptical Environmentalist: Measuring the Real State of the World*. Cambridge: Cambridge University Press.

Lopez, Barry. 1990. *The Rediscovery of North America*. Lexington, Kentucky: University Press of Kentucky.

Low, Nicholas, ed. 1999. *Global Ethics and the Environment*. New York: Routledge.

Lubchenco, Jane. 1998. Entering the Century of the Environment. *Science* 279:491–7.

Lurie, Peter; Percy Hintzen; and Robert A. Lowe. 1995. Socioeconomic Obstacles to HIV Prevention and Treatment in Developing Countries: The Roles of the International Monetary Fund and the World Bank. *AIDS* 9(6):539–46.

Lyle, John Tillman. 1985. *Design for Human Ecosystems: Landscape, Land Use, and Natural Resources*. New York: Van Nostrand Reinhold.

Macklin, Ruth. 1999. A Defense of Fundamental Principles and Human Rights: A Reply to Robert Baker. *Kennedy Institute of Ethics Journal* 8(4):403–22.

Maeder, Paul; Andreas Fliessbach; David Dubois; Lucie Gunst; Padrout Fried; and Urs Niggle. 2002. Soil Fertility and Biodiversity in Organic Farming. *Science*:1694–7.

Margalit, Avishai; translated by Naomi Goldblum. 1996. *The Decent Society*. Cambridge: Harvard University Press.

Marietta, Don E., Jr.; and Lester Embree, eds. 1995. *Environmental Philosophy and Environmental Activism*. Lanham, Maryland: Rowman & Littlefield.

Mariner, Wendy K. 1995. Rationing Health Care and the Need for Credible Scarcity: Why Americans Can't Say No. *American Journal of Public Health* 85(10):1439–45.

Marmot, Michael. 2002. The Influence of Income on Health: Views of an Epidemiologist. *Health Affairs* 21(2):31–46.

Marsh, George Perkins. 1898. *The Earth as Modified by Human Action: A Last Revision of "Man and Nature."* New York: C. Scribner.

Marshall, Peter. 1994. *Nature's Web: Rethinking Our Place on Earth*. New York: Paragon House.

Maxwell, R. J. 1985. Resource Constraints and the Quality of Care. *Lancet* 2(8461): 936–9.

Mazur, Laurie Ann. 1994. *Beyond the Numbers: A Reader on Population, Consumption and Environment*. Washington, D.C.: Island Press.

McCally, Michael. 2000. Environment and Health: An Overview. *Canadian Medical Association Journal* 163(5):533–5.

McCally, Michael, ed. 2002. *Life Support: The Environment and Human Health*. Cambridge: MIT Press.

McCally, Michael; and Christine K. Cassel. 1990. Medical Responsibility and Global Environmental Change. *Annals of Internal Medicine*. 113(6):467–73.

McDonough, William; and Michael Braungart. 2002. *Cradle to Cradle: Remaking the Way We Make Things*. New York: North Point Press.

McGee, Glenn. 1997. *The Perfect Baby: A Pragmatic Approach to Genetics*. Lanham, Maryland: Rowman & Littlefield.

———, ed. 1999. *Pragmatic Bioethics*. Nashville: Vanderbilt University Press.

McKenzie, Dorothy. 1991. *Design for the Environment*. New York: Rizzoli.

McKeown, Thomas. 1979. *The Role of Medicine: Dream, Mirage, or Nemesis?* Princeton: Princeton University Press.

McMichael, Anthony J. 1993. *Planetary Overload: Global Environmental Change and the Health of the Human Species*. Cambridge: Cambridge University Press.

———. 1994. Global Environmental Change and Human Health: New Challenges to Scientist and Policy Maker. *Journal of Public Health Policy* 15(4):407–19.

———. 1995. Global Climate Change and Health. *Lancet* 346:835.

———. 2001. *Human Frontiers, Environments, and Disease*. Cambridge: Cambridge University Press.

McMichael, Anthony; Anthony Haines; R Slooff; and S. Kovats, eds. 1996. *Climate Change and Human Health*. Geneva: World Health Organization.

McMichael, Anthony J.; Alistair J. Woodward; and Ruud E. van Leeuwen. 1994. The Impact of Energy Use in Industrialized Countries upon Global Population Health. *Medicine & Global Survival* 1: 23–32.

McNeill, John R. 2001. *Something New under the Sun: An Environmental History of the Twentieth-century World*. New York: W. W. Norton & Company.

Meadows, Donella H.; Dennis L. Meadows; Jørgen Randers; and William W. Behrens III. 1972. *Limits to Growth: A Report for the Club of Rome's Project on the Predicament of Mankind*. New York: Universe Books.

Meadows, Donella H.; Dennis L. Meadows; and Jørgen Randers. 1992. *Beyond the Limits: Confronting Global Collapse, Envisioning a Sustainable Future*. Post Mills, Vermont: Chelsea Green.

Mehlman, Maxwell J. 1991. The Oregon Medicaid Program: Is It Just? *Health Matrix* 1(2):175–99.

Merchant, Carolyn. 1985. *The Death of Nature: Women, Ecology, and the Scientific Revolution*. San Francisco: Harper & Row.

Meyer, William B. 1996. *Human Impact on the Earth*. Cambridge, U.K.: Cambridge University Press.

Mitcham, Carl. 1996. Biomedical Technologies and the Environment: Rejecting the Ethics of Rejecting Nature. In *The Ecology of Health: Identifying Issues and Alternatives*. Edited by Jennifer Chesworth. Thousand Oaks, California: Sage Publications.

Mitka, Mike. 2001. Relate Global Health to Policy, Says Report. *Journal of the American Medical Association* 286(10):1164.

Moeller, Dade. 1997. *Environmental Health*. Revised ed. Cambridge: Harvard University Press.

Mollison, Bill. 1990. *Permaculture: A Practical Guide for a Sustainable Future*. Washington, D.C.: Island Press.

Monagle, John F.; and David C. Thomasma, eds. 1998. *Health Care Ethics: Critical Issues for the 21st Century*. Gaithersburg, Maryland: Aspen Publishers.

Montague, Peter. 2003. *Mercury—How Much Is Safe?* Rachel's Health and Environment Weekly, #597, 1998 [accessed January 3, 2003]. Available from www.monitor.net/rachel/rehw-home.html.

Moore, Gary S. 1999. *Living with the Earth: Concepts in Environmental Health Science*. Boca Raton, Florida: Lewis Publishers.

Morreim, E. Haavi. 1995. *Balancing Act: The New Medical Ethics of Medicine's New Economics*. Washington, D.C.: Georgetown University Press.

Morris, David B. 1996. Environment: The White Noise of Health. *Literature and Medicine* 15(1):1–15.

———. 2002. Light as Environment: Medicine, Health, and Values. *Journal of Medical Humanities* 23(1):7–30.

Murray, Christopher J. L.; and Alan D. Lopez. 1996a. Evidence-Based Health Policy—Lessons from the Global Burden of Disease Study. *Science* 274:740–3.

Murray, Christopher J. L.; and Alan D. Lopez, eds. 1996b. *The Global Burden of Disease Study: A Comprehensive Assessment of Mortality and Disability from Diseases, Injuries, and Risk Factors in 1990 and Projected to 2020*. Cambridge: Harvard School of Public Health, on behalf of the World Health Organization and the World Bank, distributed by Harvard University Press.

Mutz, Kathryn M.; Gary C. Bryner; and Douglas S. Kenney, eds. 2002. *Justice and Natural Resouces: Concepts, Strategies, and Applications*. Washington, D.C.: Island Press.

Myers, Norman. 1995. Environmental Unknowns. *Science* 269:358–60.

Myers, Nancy; Michael Lerner; Carolyn Raffensperger; Tracy Easthope; Andrew Jameton; Ted Schettler, et al. 2002. *What Is Ecological Medicine?* Bolinas, California: The Commonweal Foundation.

Naess, Arne. 1989. *Ecology, Community, and Lifestyle*. Translated by David Rothenberg. Cambridge: Cambridge University Press.

Nash, Roderick. 1982. *Wilderness and the American Mind*. Third ed. New Haven: Yale University Press.

National Association of Physicians for the Environment. 1999. *Leadership Conference: Biomedical Research and the Environment*. Natcher Center, National Institutes of Health, Bethesda, Maryland. Nov 1–2.

National Cancer Institute Cancer Facts. 2002. *Taxanes in Cancer Treatment* [accessed November 24, 2002]. Available from cis.nci.nih.gov/fact/7_15.htm.

National Institute of Environmental Health Science. 2003. *Environmental Genome Project*. [accessed January 4, 2003]. Available from www.niehs.nih.gov/envgenom/egp.htm.

National Toxicology Program–Center for the Evaluation of Risks to Human Reproduction. 2000. NTP–CERHR Expert Panel Report on Di(2-ethylhexyl)phthalate: U.S. Department of Health and Human Services.

Natrass, Brian; and Mary Altomare. 1999. *The Natural Step for Business: Wealth, Ecology, and the Evolutionary Corporation.* Gabriola Island, British Columbia: New Society Publishers.

Neurath, Paul. 1994. *From Malthus to the Club of Rome and Back: Problems of Limits to Growth, Population Control, and Migrations.* Armonk, New York: M.E. Sharpe.

Niesink, R. J. M.; J. de Vries; and M. A. Hollinger. 1996. *Toxicology.* Boca Raton, Florida: CRC Press.

Norton, Bryan G. 1991. *Toward Unity Among Environmentalists.* New York: Oxford University Press.

―――. 1996. Moral Naturalism and Adaptive Management. *Hastings Center Report* 26(6):24–6.

Notestein, Frank W. 1945. Population—The Long View. In *Food for the World*, edited by T. W. Schultz. Chicago: University of Chicago Press.

Nuland, Sherwin B. 1994. *How We Die: Reflections on Life's Final Chapter.* New York: Alfred A. Knopf.

Nussbaum, Martha; and Amartya Sen, eds. 1993. *The Quality of Life.* New York: Oxford University Press.

Ogden, Cynthia L.; Katherine M. Flegal; Margaret D. Carroll; and Clifford L. Johnson. 2002. Prevalence and Trends in Overweight among U.S. Children and Adolescents, 1999–2000. *Journal of the American Medical Association* 288(14):1728–32.

Olshansky, S. Jay; Bruce A. Carnes; and Christine Cassel. 1990. In Search of Methuselah: Estimating the Upper Limits to Human Longevity. *Science* 250:634–40.

Onoge, Omafume F. 1975. Capitalism and Public Health: A Neglected Theme in the Medical Anthropology of Africa. In *Topias and Utopias in Health: Policy Studies*, edited by S. R. Ingman and A. E. Thomas. The Hague: Mouton.

Park, Chris. 1997. *The Environment: Principles and Applications.* New York: Routledge.

Passmore, John. 1974. *Man's Responsibility for Nature: Ecological Problems and Western Traditions.* New York: Scribner.

Patz, J. A.; Paul R. Epstein; T. A. Burke; and J. M. Balbus. 1996. Global Climate Change and Emerging Infectious Diseases. *Journal of the American Medical Association* 275:217–23.

Pearce, D.; and R. K. Turner. 1990. *Economics of Natural Resources and the Environment.* London: Harvester.

Pedersen, Duncan. 1996. Disease Ecology at a Crossroads: Man-Made Environments, Human Rights and Perpetual Development Utopias. *Social Science and Medicine.* 43(5):745–58.

Peet, John. 1992. *Energy and the Ecological Economics of Sustainability.* Washington, D.C.: Island Press.

Peterson, William. 1999. *Malthus: Founder of Modern Demography.* New Brunswick, New Jersey: Transaction Publishers.

Pierce, Jessica. 2002. Can Bioethics Survive in a Dying World? *Journal of Medical Humanities* 23(1):3–6.

Pierce, Jessica; and Christina Kerby. 1999. The Global Ethics of Latex Gloves: Reflections on Natural Resource Use in Health Care. *Cambridge Quarterly of Healthcare Ethics* 8(1):98–107.

Pierce, Jessica; Hilde Lindeman Nelson; and Karen Warren. 2002. Feminist Slants on Nature and Health. *Journal of Medical Humanities* 23(1):61–72.

Pierce, Roger. 2002. Natural Piety. *Journal of Medical Humanities* 23(1):87–92.

Pimentel, David R.; Rebecca Harman; Matthew Pacenza; Jasonn Pecarsky; and Marcia

Pimentel. 1986. Natural Resources and an Optimum Human Population. *Population and Environment* 15(5):347–69.

Pimentel, David; Maria Tort; Linda D'Anna; Anne Krawic; Joshua Berger; Jessica Rossman; Fridah Mugo; Nancy Doon; Michael Shriberg; Erica Howard; Susan Lee; and Jonathan Talbot. 1998. Ecology of Increasing Disease: Population Growth and Environmental Degradation. *Bioscience.* 48(10):817–26.

Pollack, Robert. 1999. *The Missing Moment: How the Unconscious Shapes Modern Science.* Boston: Houghton Mifflin.

Ponting, Clive. 1991. *A Green History of the World.* New York: St. Martin's Press.

Pope, C. Arden, III; Richard T. Burnett; Michael J. Thun; Eugenia E. Calle; Daniel Krewski; Ito Kazuhiko; and George D. Thurston. 2002. Lung Cancer, Cardiopulmonary Mortality, and Long-term Exposure to Fine Particulate Air Pollution. *Journal of the American Medical Association* 287(9):1132–41.

Potter, Van Rensselaer. 1971. *Bioethics: Bridge to the Future.* Englewood Cliffs, New Jersey: Prentice-Hall, Inc.

———. 1988. *Global Bioethics: Building on the Leopold Legacy.* East Lansing, Michigan: Michigan State University Press.

———. 1990. Getting to the Year 3000: Can Global Bioethics Overcome Evolution's Fatal Flaw? *Perspectives in Biology and Medicine* 34(1):89–98.

———. 1999. Fragmented Ethics and "Bridge Bioethics." *Hastings Center Report* 29(1):38–40.

Potter, Van Rensselaer; and Lisa Potter. 1995. Forum: Global Bioethics: Converting Sustainable Development to Global Survival. *Medicine and Global Survival* 2(3):185–91.

Potter, Van Rensselaer; and Peter J. Whitehouse. 1998. Deep and Global Bioethics for a Livable World. *The Scientist* 12:9.

Price, David. 1995. Energy and Human Evolution. *Population and Environment: A Journal of Interdisciplinary Studies* 16(4):301–19.

Priester, Reinhard. 1992. A Values Framework for Health System Reform. *Health Affairs* 11(2):84–107.

Princen, Thomas; Michael Maniates; and Ken Conca, eds. 2002. *Confronting Consumption.* Cambridge: MIT Press.

Proctor, Robert N. 1994. The Politics of Cancer. *Dissent* 41(2):215–22.

———. 1995. *Cancer Wars: What We Know and Don't Know About Cancer.* New York: Basic Books.

Quammen, David. 1998. Planet of Weeds: Tallying the Losses of Earth's Animals and Plants. *Harper's Magazine.* 1998 October: 57–69.

Raffensperger, Carolyn; Joel Tickner; and Wes Jackson, eds. 1999. *Protecting Public Health and the Environment: Implementing the Precautionary Principle.* Washington, D.C.: Island Press.

Ramsey, Paul. 1970. *The Patient as Person: Explorations in Medical Ethics.* New Haven: Yale University Press.

Rasmussen, Larry L. 1996. *Earth Community, Earth Ethics.* Maryknoll, New York: Orbis Books.

Rawls, John. 1971. *A Theory of Justice.* Cambridge: The Belknap Press of Harvard University Press.

Rees, J. 1990. *Natural Resources: Allocation, Economics, and Policy.* London: Routledge.

Regan, Tom. 1984. *The Case for Animal Rights.* Berkeley: University of California Press.

Reich, Warren Thomas. 1995. The Word "Bioethics": The Struggle over Its Earliest Meanings. *Kennedy Institute of Ethics Journal.* 5(1):19–34.

Reijnders, Lucas. 1998. The Factor X Debate. *Journal of Industrial Ecology* 2(1):13–22.

Richardson, Henry. 1990. Specifying Norms as a Way to Resolve Concrete Ethical Problems. *Philosophy and Public Affairs* 19(4):279–310.

———. 1995. Beyond Good and Right: Toward a Constructive Ethical Pragmatism. *Philosophy and Public Affairs* 24(2):108–41.

Rodger, Allan. 2001. Constructing Sustainable Futures: Towards Self-Organizing Communities. In *Ecospheres: Papers*, edited by C. Steward and C. McGuire. Lincoln, Nebraska: University of Nebraska and Joslyn Castle Institute for Sustainable Communities.

Rolston III, Holmes. 1988. *Environmental Ethics*. Philadelphia: Temple University Press.

———. 1996. Feeding People Versus Saving Nature. In *World Hunger and Morality*, edited by W. Aiken and H. LaFollette. Upper Saddle River, New Jersey: Prentice Hall.

Rosenblatt, Robert. 1995. Introduction to Rescue: The Paradoxes of Virtue. *Social Research.* 62(1):3–6.

Rutala, William; Robert L. Odette; and Gregory Samsa. 1989. Management of Infectious Waste by U.S. Hospitals. *Journal of the American Medical Association* 262(12):1635–40.

Ryan, John C.; Alan Thein Durning; and Don Baker. 1997. *Stuff: The Secret Lives of Everyday Things*. Seattle: Northwest Environment Watch.

Sachs, Aaron. 1995. *Eco-Justice: Linking Human Rights and the Environment, Worldwatch Paper 127*. Washington, D.C.: Worldwatch Institute.

———. 1996. Upholding Human Rights and Environmental Justice. In *State of the World 1996: A Worldwatch Institute Report on Progress Toward a Sustainable Society*, edited by L. R. Brown. New York: W. W. Norton & Company.

Sagoff, Mark. 1997. Do We Consume Too Much? *The Atlantic Monthly*, 80–96.

Saito, Yuriko. 2002. Ecological Design: Promises and Challenges. *Environmental Ethics* 24(3):243–61.

Salgado, Sebastião et al. 1993. Introduction. In *Workers: An Archeaology of the Industrial Age*, edited by S. Salgado. New York: Aperture.

Scheper-Hughes, Nancy.1992. *Death Without Weeping*. Berkeley: University of California Press.

Schmidt, Charles W. 2002. More at Stake Than Steak. *Environmental Health Perspectives* 110(7):A396–A402.

Scholte, Jan Aart. 2000. *Globalization*. New York: St. Martin's Press.

Schultz, Theodore W. 1945. *Food for the World*. Chicago: University of Chicago Press.

Sen, Amartya. 1997. *On Economic Inequality*. Enlarged ed. Oxford: Clarendon Press.

Shi, Leiyu; and Douglas Singh. 1998. *Delivering Health Care in America: A Systems Approach*. Gaithersburg, Maryland: Aspen Publishers, Inc.

Shiva, Vandana. 1989. *Staying Alive: Women, Ecology and Development*. London: Zed Books Ltd.

Shrader-Frechette, Kristin. 1991. Ethics and the Environment. *World Health Forum* 12:311–21.

Siddiqi, Javed. 1995. *World Health and World Politics: The World Health Organization and the U.N. System*. Columbia: University of South Carolina Press.

Sikdar, S. K; and M. El-Halwagi. 2001. *Process Design Tools for the Environment*. London: Taylor & Francis.

Simbruner, George. 1993. Ecological Impact of Pediatric Intensive Care. *Critical Care Medicine* 21(9[supplement]):S399.

Simmons, I. G. 1993. *Interpreting Nature: Cultural Constructions of the Environment*. London: Routledge.

Simon, Julian; and Herman Kahn. 1984. *The Resourceful Earth*. Oxford: Basil Blackwell.

Singer, Peter. 1975. *Animal Liberation*. New York: A New York Review Book.

———. 1996. Famine, Affluence, and Morality. In *World Hunger and Morality*, edited by W. Aiken and H. LaFollette. Upper Saddle River, New Jersey: Prentice Hall.

———. 2000. *A Darwinian Left: Politics, Evolution, and Cooperation*. New Haven: Yale University Press.

———. 2002. *One World: The Ethics of Globalization*. New Haven: Yale University Press.

Sinsheimer, Robert L. 1978. The Presumptions of Science. *Daedalus* 107(2):23–35.

Smil, Vaclav. 1991. Population Growth and Nitrogen: An Exploration of a Critical Essential Link. *Population and Development Review* 17(4):569–601.

———. 1994a. *Energy and World History*. Boulder, Colorado: Westview Press.

———. 1994b. How Many People Can the Earth Feed. *Population and Development Review* 20(2):255–92.

———. 1997. Global Population and the Nitrogen Cycle. *Scientific American* July:76–81.

———. 2000. *Feeding the World: A Challenge for the Twenty-first Century*. Cambridge: MIT Press.

Snow, C. P. 1993. *The Two Cultures*. Reissue ed. Cambridge: Cambridge University Press.

Soejarto, D. D. 1996. Biodiversity Prospecting and Benefit-Sharing: Perspectives from the Field. *Journal of Ethnopharmacology* 51(1–3):1–15.

Solomon, Gina M.; and Ted Schettler. 2000. Environment and Health: 6. Endocrine Disruption and Potential Human Health Impacts. *Canadian Medical Association Journal* 163(11):1471–6.

Somerville, Margaret A. 1995. Planet as Patient. *Ecosystem Health* 1(2):61–71.

Soper, Kate. 1995. *What Is Nature?: Culture, Politics and the Non-Human*. Cambridge: Blackwell.

Speidel, Joseph. 2000. Environment and Health: 1. Population, Consumption and Human Health. *Canadian Medical Association Journal* 163(5):551–6.

Steingraber, Sandra. 1998. *Living Downstream*. New York: Vintage Books.

Stern, Paul C.; Thomas Dietz; Vernon W. Ruttan; Robert H. Socolow; and James L. Sweeney, eds. 1997. *Environmentally Significant Consumption*. Washington, D.C.: National Academy Press.

Stocker, Karen; Howard Waitzkin; and Celia Iriart. 1999. The Exportation of Managed Care to Latin America. *New England Journal of Medicine* 340(14): 1131–6.

Strosberg, Martin A.; Joshua M. Weiner; Robert Baker; and I. Alan Fein. 1992. Rationing America's Medical Care: the Oregon Plan and Beyond. Washington, D.C.: The Brookings Institute.

Takala, Tuija. 2001. What Is Wrong with Global Bioethics? On the Limitations of the Four Principles Approach. *Cambridge Quarterly of Healthcare Ethics* 10(1):72–7.

Tarkan, Laurie. 2001. Research Is Urged for Healthier Breast Milk. *The New York Times*, October 16, p. D6.

Taylor, Paul W. 1986. *Respect for Nature: A Theory of Environmental Ethics*. Princeton: Princeton University Press.

———. 1998. The Ethics of Respect for Nature. In *The Environmental Ethics and Policy Book*, edited by Donald VanDeVeer and Christine Pierce. Belmont, California: Wadsworth.

Taxolog, Inc. 2000–2001. *The Taxol Story* [accessed November 24, 2002]. Available at www.taxolog.com/taxol.html.

Thomas, Keith. 1996. *Man and the Natural World: Changing Attitudes in England, 1500–1800*. New York: Oxford University Press.

Thornton, Joe. 2000. *Pandora's Poison: Chlorine, Health, and a New Environmental Strategy*. Cambridge: MIT Press.

Tieszen, M. E.; and J. C. Gruenberg. 1992. A Quantitative, Qualitative, and Critical Assessment of Surgical Waste. Surgeons Venture Through the Trash Can. *Journal of the American Medical Association* 267(20): 2765–8.

Timmermann, A.; J. Oberhuber; A. Bacher; M. Esch; M. Latif; and E. Roeckner. 1999. Increased El Niño Frequency in a Climate Model Forced by Future Greenhouse Warming. *Nature* 398:694–7.

Todd, Nancy Jack; and John Todd. 1994. *From Eco-Cities to Living Machines: Principles of Ecological Design*. Berkeley: North Atlantic Books.

Toebes, Brigit C. A. 1999. *The Right to Health as a Human Right in International Law*. Edited by C. Flinterman, *School of Human Rights Research Series*. Antwerp, Belgium: Intersentia.

Torrance, Robert M., ed. 1998. *Encompassing Nature: A Sourcebook*. Washington, D.C.: Counterpoint.

Toulmin, Stephen. 1982. How Medicine Saved the Life of Ethics. *Perspectives in Biology and Medicine* 25(4):736–50.

U.S. Bureau of the Census, Report WP/98. 1999. *World Population Profile: 1998*. Washington, D.C.: U.S. Government Printing Office.

Ubel, Peter A. 2000. *Pricing Life: Why It's Time for Health Care Rationing*. Cambridge: MIT Press.

Union of Concerned Scientists. 1992. *World Scientists' Warning to Humanity*. Cambridge: Union of Concerned Scientists.

United Nations. 2000. *World Population Prospects: The 2000 Revision*, Highlights. [accessed March 24, 2003]. Available from www.un.org/esa/population/wpp2000/highlights/df.

United Nations Development Programme. 2000. *World Energy Assessment*. New York: United Nations Development Programme.

United Nations Development Programme, United Nations Environment Programme, World Bank, and World Resources Institute. 2000. *A Guide to World Resources 2000–2001: People and Ecosystems, The Fraying Web of Life*. Washington, D.C.: World Resources Institute.

United Nations Development Programme, United Nations Department of Economic and Social Affairs, World Energy Council. 2000b. *World Energy Assessment*. New York: United Nations Development Programme.

United Nations Environment Programme. 2001. *Global Environment Outlook—2000* [accessed January 5, 2003]. Available at http://www.grida.no/geo2000/.

———. 2002. *Global Environment Outlook 3*. London: Earthscan.

United Nations Environment Programme, United Nations Children's Fund, and World Health Organization. 2002. *Children in the New Millenium: Environmental Impact on Health*. Geneva: World Health Organization.

United Nations Population Fund. 2002. *The State of the World's Population* 2001 [accessed May 5 2002]. Available from www.unfpa.org/swp/2001.

United States Committee for Refugees. 2002. *World Refugee Survey 2002*. Washington, D.C.: United States Committee for Refugees.

Van der Ryn, Sim; and Stuart Cowan. 1996. *Ecological Design*. Washington, D.C.: Island Press.

VanDeVeer, Donald; and Christine Pierce, eds. 1998. *The Environmental Ethics and Policy Book*. Second ed. Belmont, California: Wadsworth.

Varner, Gary E. 1998. *In Nature's Interest? Interests, Animal Rights, and Environmental Ethics*. New York: Oxford University Press.

Veatch, Robert M. 2000. *The Basics of Bioethics*. Upper Saddle River, New Jersey: Prentice Hall.

Vitousek, Peter M. 1994. Beyond Global Warming Ecology and Global Change. *Ecology* 75(7):1861–76.

Vitousek, Peter M.; Paul R. Ehrlich; Anne H. Ehrlich; and Pamela A. Matson. 1986. Human Appropriation of the Products of Biosynthesis. *BioScience* 34(6):368–73.

Vitousek, Peter M.; Harold A. Mooney; Jane Lubchenco; and Jerry M. Melillo. 1997. Human Domination of Earth's Ecosystems. *Science* 277:494–9.

Wackernagel, Mathis; and William Rees. 1996. *Our Ecological Footprint: Reducing Human Impact on the Earth*. Philadelphia: New Society Publishers.

Wackernagel, Mathis; Niels B. Schulz; Diana Deumling; Alejandro Callejas Linares; Martin Jenkins; Valerie Kapos; Chad Monfreda; Jonathan Loh; Norman Myers; Richard Norgaard; and Jørgen Randers. 2002. Tracking the Ecological Overshoot of the Human Economy. *Proceedings of the National Academy of Sciences* 99(14): 9266–71.

Walt, Gill. 1998. Globalization of International Health. *Lancet* 351:434–7.

Walter, Jonathan, principal contributor. 2002. *World Disasters Report 2002*. [accessed 20 November 2002]. Available from www.ifrc.org.

Walther, G. R. et al. 2002. Ecological Responses to Recent Climate Change. *Nature* 416(6879):389–95.

Wear, Stephen; James J. Bono; Gerald Logue; and Adrianne McEvoy, eds. 2000. *Ethical Issues in Health Care on the Frontiers of the Twenty-first Century*. Dordrecht, The Netherlands: Kluwer Academic Publishers.

von Weizsäcker, Ernst Ulrich; Amory B. Lovins; and L. Hunter Lovins. 1997. *Factor Four: Doubling Wealth, Halving Resource Use*. London: Earthscan Publications, Ltd.

Wennberg, John E.; Elliot S. Fisher; and Jonathan S. Skinner. 2002. Geography and the Debate over Medicare Reform. *Health Affairs*:W96–W114.

Wernick, Iddo K. 1996. Consuming Materials: The American Way. *Technological Forecasting and Social Change*. 53:111–22.

Wernick, Iddo K.; Robert Herman; Skekhar Govind; and Jesse Ausubel. 1996. Materialization and Dematerialization: Measures and Trends. *Daedalus* 125(3):171–98.

Weston, Anthony. 1992. *Toward Better Problems*. Philadelphia: Temple University Press.

Westra, Laura; and Patricia H. Werhane, eds. 1998. *The Business of Consumption*. Lanham, Maryland: Rowman & Littlefield, Inc.

Westra, Laura; and Peter S. Wenz. 1995. *Faces of Environmental Racism*. Lanham, Maryland: Rowman & Littlefield.

White, Lynn, Jr. 1967. The Historical Roots of Our Ecological Crisis. *Science* (March 10).

Whitehouse, Peter J. 1999. The Ecomedical Disconnection Syndrome. *Hastings Center Report*. 29(1):41–44.

Whittaker, R. H.; and G. E. Likens. 1975. The Biosphere and Man. In *Primary Productivity and the Biosphere*, edited by H. Leith and R. H. Whittaker. Berlin: Springer-Verlag.

Wilkinson, Richard G. 1992. Income Distribution and Life Expectancy. *British Medical Journal* 304:165–8.

———. 1996. *Unhealthy Societies: The Afflictions of Inequality*. London: Routledge.

Wilson, Edward O. 1993. Is Humanity Suicidal? *The New York Times Magazine*. May 30; D24–D29.

World Bank. 1993. *The World Development Report 1993: Investing in Health*. Oxford: Oxford University Press.

World Commission on Environment and Development. 1987. *Our Common Future*. New York: Oxford University Press.

World Federation of Public Health Associations. 2002. *WFPHA Policy Resolutions and Position Papers 2001* [accessed December 29 2002]. Available from www.apha.org/wfpha/policy.htm.

World Health Organization. 1978. *Primary Health Care: Report of the International Conference on Primary Health Care, Alma-Ata, USSR, 6–12 September 1978.* Geneva: World Health Organization.

———. 1992. *Our Planet, Our Health: Report of the WHO Commission on Health and Environment.* Geneva: World Health Organization.

———. 2000. *World Health Report—2000: Health Systems: Improving Performance.* Geneva, Switzerland: World Health Organization.

World Health Organization, Advisory Committee on Health Research. 2002. Genomics and World Health: Report of the Advisory Committee on Health Research. Geneva: World Health Organization.

World Wildlife Fund. 1999. *Living Planet Report 1999.* Gland, Switzerland: World Wide Fund for Nature.

———. 2002. *Living Planet Report 2002.* Gland, Switzerland: World Wide Fund for Nature.

Worldwatch Institute. 2001. *State of the World 2001.* Edited by L. Brown, C. Flavin, and H. French. New York: W. W. Norton & Company.

Wright, Michaella; and Bruce Maine. 2001. Sustainable Design. In *Creating Responsive Solutions to Healthcare Change*, edited by C. S. McCollough. Indianapolis: Center Nursing Press.

Yach, Derek. 1996. Tobacco in Africa. *World Health Forum* 17(1):29–36.

Yach, D.; and D. Bettcher. 1998. The Globalization of Public Health, I: Threats and Opportunities. *American Journal of Public Health* 88(5):738–41.

Yoon, Carol Kaesuk. 2001. Struggle to Survive for an "Urban Whale." *The New York Times,* October 16, D4.

Zimmerman, Michael E.; ed. by J. Baird Callicott; George Sessions; Karen J. Warren; and John Clark. 1998. *Environmental Philosophy: From Animal Rights to Radical Ecology.* Second ed. Upper Saddle River, New Jersey: Prentice Hall.

Index